CONCISE GUIDE TO

Geriatric Psychiatry

American Psychiatric Press

CONCISE GUIDES

Robert E. Hales, M.D.
Series Editor

CONCISE GUIDE TO

GERIATRIC PSYCHIATRY

James E. Spar, M.D.

Associate Clinical Professor
Department of Psychiatry and Biobehavioral Sciences
Coordinator, Clinical Geriatric Services
Neuropsychiatric Institute and Hospital
University of California, Los Angeles

Asenath La Rue, Ph.D.

Associate Professor in Residence
Department of Psychiatry and Biobehavioral Sciences
Neuropsychiatric Institute and Hospital
University of California, Los Angeles

American
Psychiatric
Press, Inc.

Washington, DC
London, England

The paper used in this publication meets the minimum require-
ments of the American National Standard for Information Sciences—Permanence of Paper for Printed Library Materials,
ANSI Z39.48-1984.   ∞

American Psychiatric Press, Inc.
1400 K Street, NW
Washington, D.C. 20005

Library of Congress Cataloging-in-Publication Data
Spar, James E.
    Concise guide to geriatric psychiatry / James E. Spar,
Asenath La Rue. —1st ed.
        p.   cm.—(Concise guides / American Psychiatric
Press)
    Includes bibliographical references.
    ISBN 0-88048-335-0 (alk. paper)
    1. Geriatric psychiatry.   I. La Rue, Asenath, 1948-
II. Title.   III. Series: Concise guides (American Psychiatric
Press)
        [DNLM: 1. Mental Disorders—in old age.   WT 150
        S736c]
    RC451.4.A5S67   1990
    618.97′689—dc20
    DNLM/DLC
    for Library of Congress   89-18625
                                                        CIP

British Cataloguing in Publication Data
A CIP record is available from the British Library.

This book is dedicated to Dr. Jolly West
and to the memories of Drs. Henry Lesse, Phillip May,
and Richard Walter.

CONTENTS

INTRODUCTION

to the *American Psychiatric Press Concise Guides*

The *American Psychiatric Press Concise Guides* series provides, in a most accessible format, practical information for psychiatrists—and especially for psychiatry residents and medical students—working in such varied treatment settings as inpatient psychiatry services, outpatient clinics, consultation-liaison services, and private practice. The *Concise Guides* are meant to complement the more detailed information to be found in lengthier psychiatry texts.

The *Concise Guides* address topics of greatest concern to psychiatrists in clinical practice. The books in this series contain a detailed table of contents, along with an index, tables, and charts, for easy access; and their size, designed to fit into a lab coat pocket, makes them a convenient source of information. The number of references has been limited to those most relevant to the material presented.

With the increased number of senior citizens in the United States, geriatric psychiatry has become an important psychiatry subspecialty. Drs. James E. Spar and Asenath La Rue are experts in this field. Both are Associate Professors in the Department of Psychiatry and Biobehavioral Sciences at the University of California, Los Angeles (UCLA). They have written extensively on many topics related to geriatric psychiatry and have treated a number of elderly patients as a part of the Clinical Geriatric Services at the UCLA Neuropsychiatric Institute.

They begin their book by discussing epidemiological findings that demonstrate convincingly that older people more frequently use hospital and physician services. They also provide information demonstrating that at least 12% of older adults have diagnosable mental disorders and that as many as 40–50% of elderly patients hospitalized for mental disorders may suffer from psychiatric disease. Unfortunately, as Drs. Spar and La Rue emphasize, geriatric patients frequently do not receive adequate health or mental health care. They end this introductory chapter by emphasizing how psychiatrists and other physicians may work more effectively with older patients.

Their second chapter, titled "Normal Aging," provides the reader with much important information covering the aging process. They discuss such issues as the cognitive abilities of older patients, what personality and emotional changes occur through aging, how older patients adapt to stress, and what are the implications for psychiatric treatment of various biological changes that these patients undergo. Within the framework of the normal aging process, Drs. Spar and La Rue turn their attention to the most common psychiatric disorders encountered in the elderly: mood disorders, organic mental disorders, anxiety disorders, sleep disorders, substance use disorders, sexual dysfunction, and psychiatric symptoms related to medical illness.

In their two chapters on mood disorders, the authors emphasize diagnosis and treatment. They discuss how elderly patients with major depression may present clinically in many different ways. Some patients may regress behaviorally, exhibit psychotic symptoms, have dementia-like findings, or principally complain of somatic symptoms. They provide very helpful information about laboratory tests, rating scales, and psychological tests that may assist clinicians in making the appropriate diagnosis. They also emphasize why it is important to make the proper diagnosis of major depression in these patients and how to distinguish major depression from normal bereavement, organic mood disorders, dysthymic disorder, and characterological depression. Although less common in this population, bipolar disorder is discussed, and the authors provide pertinent information concerning this diagnosis in geriatric patients.

Their chapter on the treatment of mood disorders is quite practical and clinically relevant. They discuss each of the major psychosocial therapies—individual, group, and family therapy—and a whole range of psychopharmacologic treatments such as cyclic antidepressants, monamine oxidase inhibitors, and psychostimulants. They provide excellent clinical suggestions concerning the treatment of psychotic depression and discuss how electroconvulsive therapy may be quite effective for selected patients.

Dementia and delirium are also quite common disorders in this population, especially for those who are hospitalized on medication and surgical services. Drs. Spar and La Rue provide a comprehensive summary on how psychiatrists and psychologists may work together and use appropriate tests to distinguish primary from secondary dementia and how through careful clinical assessment and a review of medications and laboratory tests, treatable causes of dementia may be identified. They provide an excellent summary of Alzheimer's disease and discuss neuropathology, neurochemistry, genetics, and other etiological considerations.

Their chapter on anxiety disorders and psychosis addresses the major clinical entities encountered in the elderly population: situational anxiety, generalized anxiety, adjustment anxiety, phobic anxiety, obsessive-compulsive disorders, and panic disorders. They also provide helpful information concerning the diagnosis and treatment of late-onset psychosis, a clinical disorder that is frequently encountered in these patients. Their final chapter discusses other common mental disorders of the elderly: sleep disorders (with a focus on insomnia), substance abuse and alcoholism, and sexual dysfunction.

There are many excellent features of this book that make it particularly outstanding for residents, medical students, and clinicians who frequently treat elderly patients who have psychiatric disorders. The authors have included over 50 outstanding tables and a number of figures that highlight important clinical material. The reader will be pleased with the clear, precise prose and the clinically relevant information throughout the book. The authors demonstrate remarkable ability to integrate complex material in a coherent and logical fashion. Readers will be pleased with the up-to-date references and the timely discussion of important clinical topics. There are a number of 1988 and 1989 references, and the authors have included selected additional readings at the end of each chapter that the reader may wish to turn to for further information and clarification.

Drs. James E. Spar and Asenath La Rue have prepared an outstanding *Concise Guide to Geriatric Psychiatry*. This wonderfully written, pocket-sized book should be of great help to psychiatrists and other mental health professionals who treat elderly patients who suffer from psychiatric disorders.

Robert E. Hales, M.D.
Series Editor
American Psychiatric Press Concise Guides

Concise Guide Series Titles

INTRODUCTION

■ CONTEMPORARY AGING AND HEALTH CARE

For the first time in history, most people in societies such as our own can plan on growing old. The average life expectancy for a woman born in the United States today is 78.2 years and for a man is 71.2 years (1). Even those who are currently "old" can expect to live many more years; for example, average life expectancy at age 65 is 18.6 years for women and 14.6 years for men.

About 21% of the current United States population is above the age of 55, and 12% is age 65 or older (1). The elderly are the only segment of the population that is expected to grow substantially in the next 50 years, so that by the year 2030, one in three Americans will be age 55 or older, and one in five at least age 65 (1). Very old people (85+ years) constitute one of the fastest growing subgroups (Figure 1-1). In 1900, there were only 123,000 people aged 85 years or older in the United States, compared to an estimated 2.2 million in 1980. By 2050, there will be 16 million people in this 85+ age group, or 5% of the total population.

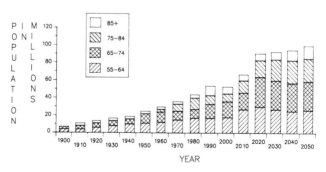

FIGURE 1-1. **Population 55 years and older, 1900–2050.**
Adapted from U.S. Senate Special Committee on Aging: Aging America—trends and projections. Washington, DC, U.S. Department of Health and Human Services, 1987–1988, p 11.

As growing old has become more predictable, health problems of the elderly have assumed a new importance. More than 80% of people age 65 and older have at least one chronic medical illness, and many have multiple conditions (1). The elderly are affected much more often than middle-aged people by arthritis and orthopedic conditions, hypertension and heart conditions, and hearing or visual impairment (Table 1-1). Each of these conditions can limit independent function and detract from quality of life. Heart disease, cancer, and stroke are the primary causes of death in the elderly and also account for many doctor visits and days of hospitalization (Figure 1-2).

Older people are hospitalized twice as often as younger adults, make more outpatient visits to physicians (in a ratio of 3:2), and use twice as many prescription drugs (1). In 1985, persons over the age of 65 accounted for 30% of all hospital discharges and 41% of all short-stay hospital days. People age 75 and above, who constitute only 5% of the current population, accounted for 16% of hospital discharges and 22% of short-stay hospital days. An average of 4 hospital discharge diagnoses are assigned to elderly patients as opposed to only 2.4 diagnoses for younger adult patients (1).

Although older people make frequent use of medical facili-

TABLE 1-1. **Common medical conditions in the elderly**

	Prevalence at ages ≥65 years (%)	Increase from condition at ages 45–64 years (%)
Arthritis	48	59
Hypertension	39	64
Hearing loss	30	46
Heart conditions	28	44
Orthopedic conditions	17	9
Diabetes	10	65
Visual impairment	10	48

Adapted from U.S. Senate Special Committee on Aging: Aging America—trends and projections. Washington, DC, U.S. Department of Health and Human Services, 1987–1988.

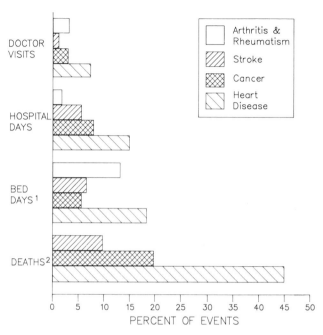

FIGURE 1-2. **Morbidity and mortality for selected conditions—ages 65 and older.**
[1]Average for 1979 and 1980. [2]Provisional data.

ties and personnel, many of their day-to-day needs for assistance with health problems are met by relatives and friends. For disabled older people living in the community, relatives provide 84% of the care; about 80% of these caregivers provide assistance on a daily basis, and 64% do so for at least a year (1).

Those with chronic needs that cannot be met at home generally receive care in nursing homes. At any given time, only about 5% of the elderly population are residing in nursing homes, but the lifetime risk for this type of institutionalization is much higher, estimated at 52% for women and 30% for men who have reached the age of 65 (1).

One-third of United States health dollars are expended on older adults, and these costs are projected to increase dramatically in the next few years (1). Per capita spending in 1984 was $4,200 per elderly person, of which 45% was spent for hospitalization, nearly 21% for physician services, and an additional 21% for nursing-home care (1).

These trends present a significant challenge to the health care community. The need to learn about aging and older people extends throughout the medical profession. Creative approaches will be required to stem rising costs while maintaining quality assessment and intervention. Alliances with families and other natural supports need to be formed to assure continuity of care, and the strengths of older patients themselves must be marshaled to cope with illness and to interact effectively within the health care system.

■ MENTAL DISORDERS IN LATER LIFE

Older people with mental disorders constitute a significant subgroup of the elderly population. At least 12% of older adults in the community have diagnosable mental disorders (2). Estimates are much higher among elderly patients hospitalized for medical conditions, where 40–50% suffer from psychiatric conditions (3,4), and in long-term care settings, between 70 and 94% of residents have been found to have mental disorders (1,5). In state mental hospitals, 27% of patients are 65 years or older (1). Overall, it is estimated that 15–25% of the 28 million Americans over the age of 65 have significant mental health problems (1).

Older patients experience the same broad spectrum of mental disorders as younger adults. However, certain conditions are particularly notable in later life, either because of increased prevalence or high morbidity (see Table 1-2).

The elderly are at much greater risk for cognitive impairment than younger adults. In the community, nearly 5% of people 65 years or older have prominent cognitive deficits, compared to less than 1% of people between the ages of 18 and 64 (2), and as many as 10–18% of older people have milder cognitive problems.

TABLE 1-2. **Mental disorders among older adults**

| Category of illness | Distribution of psychiatric diagnoses (%) | |
	Community residents[a]	Medical/surgical inpatients[b]
Cognitive impairment	4.9	30.2
Affective disorders	2.5	18.5
Anxiety disorders	5.5	5.2
Alcohol abuse/dependence	0.9	2.6
Schizophrenic disorders	0.1	0
Somatization	0.1	0
Personality disorder	0	8.3
Other psychiatric disorder	0	7.9

[a]Adapted from Regier DA, Boyd JH, Burke JD, et al: One-month prevalence of mental disorders in the United States. Arch Gen Psychiatry 45:977–986, 1988.
[b]Adapted from Rapp SR, Parisi SA, Walsh DA: Psychological dysfunction and physical health among elderly medical inpatients. J Consult Clin Psychol 56:851–855, 1988.

In medical hospital settings, between one-third and one-half of elderly patients have either transient or persistent cognitive impairment (3,4).

Cognitive deficits in older patients have many different possible causes, and in about one patient in five, treatment of underlying problems can reverse or substantially alleviate cognitive symptoms (6). Even for patients with dementia of the Alzheimer type, gains in functional ability can be obtained by treating coexisting medical or psychiatric illnesses (7). These small gains can make a great difference to family members caring for these patients, as can support, psychotherapy, and respite provided for caregivers.

Depression is an equally important condition in older adults. In the community, the percentages of older people meeting strict diagnostic criteria for major depression or dysthymic disorder are quite low (0.7 and 1.85%, respectively, over 6 months) (2). However, traditional diagnostic criteria do not do justice to the prevalence of depressive symptoms among older people (8,9). At least 8% of elderly community residents have serious depressive symptoms, and nearly 19% have less severe dysphoric symptomatology (8). In addition, in medical hospitals, at least one-quarter of older patients have diagnosable mood disorders (3,4), and nearly one-half of the admissions of older adults to psychiatric hospitals are for depressive conditions (9).

Geriatric depression can be treated effectively with standard therapies, but is unlikely to resolve spontaneously. Certain subgroups of older patients, especially Caucasian men, are at very high risk for suicide (1), increasing the importance of accurately detecting and treating geriatric depression.

Many older people without major mental disorders experience adjustment reactions to personal stresses, bereavement, pain syndromes, and sleep disturbance. Education and interventions directed at these problems may prevent more serious psychiatric or medical problems from developing.

For psychiatrists, then, there are at least two important roles to fill for older patients. The first is to identify and treat specific psychiatric disorders. The second is to provide education, support, and preventive interventions to strengthen older people and their families in managing common stresses of aging.

■ BARRIERS TO GERIATRIC MENTAL HEALTH CARE

There is general consensus that older people are poorly served by the mental health system (10). Only about 5% of psychiatrists' clinical hours are spent with older patients, and only 6% of the clientele at community mental health centers are over the age of 65 (10). Overall, it is estimated that only a small fraction of elderly persons receive the mental health services warranted by their conditions (11).

The gap between needs and services has many causes. The most tangible, and probably the most important, are limited reimbursement, limited access, and staffing patterns (10–12). Attitudes also play a role, as does limited training in geriatric psychiatry.

Psychiatrists and other mental health specialists may find it difficult to work with elderly patients. Understandably, they often prefer to work with patients or clients who have less daunting problems with physical illness and personal loss, who remind them less of their own mortality, and who are less likely to die in the course of treatment. Nonetheless, recent research has not found health care professionals to be strongly or pervasively negative in their attitudes about older patients (12). Instead, age bias seems to take more specific forms. For example, American psychiatrists and other mental health workers tend to overdiagnose organic mental disorders in the elderly (9,12) and tend to refer older patients less often for psychotherapy than comparably ill younger clients (12,13). There is also a growing concern that ageism may be assuming new forms. Some professionals, in an attempt to avoid discrimination against the elderly, may exaggerate the competencies and excuse the deficits of elderly patients (12).

Elderly people themselves contribute to inadequate mental health care. Most are likely to consult other medical specialists, such as their family doctor or an internist, instead of seeking a psychiatrist's services. Current cohorts of older people focus heavily on the reporting of physical symptoms as opposed to psychological events, and if psychological complaints are raised, they are most often communicated to a primary-care physician (14).

Unfortunately, in medical settings, mental disorders are generally overlooked when psychiatric input is not available (15). This problem is particularly common for elderly patients (4,15). There are many reasons why this may be so. The elderly rely more heavily than younger patients on primary-care physicians; their multiple medical illnesses may divert physicians' attention away from psychiatric signs and symptoms; depression and anxiety may be viewed as normal for older people with serious medical illness; and physicians with neither psychiatric nor geriatric training may find it hard to distinguish normal aging changes from signs of mental disorder. In one recent study (16), medical residents were found to be aware of the possibility of comorbid depression in elderly patients and strongly motivated to detect and treat depressive symptoms; however, their knowledge of basic diagnostic criteria was so limited that they detected fewer than 10% of cases of clinically significant depression among older medical or surgical patients.

There is, therefore, a clear need for psychiatrists to be willing to work with the elderly, both in primary-care and consultation roles. This work is needed in psychiatric and medical hospitals, health maintenance organizations, community mental health centers, private practice, and long-term care.

■ WORKING EFFECTIVELY WITH OLDER PATIENTS

Psychiatric care of older patients requires a blending of specialized knowledge with a broadly based, flexible approach to the patient (Table 1-3).

In addition to mastering the content areas covered in this Concise Guide, certain personal qualities and professional approaches are important for effective work in geriatric psychiatry (Table 1-4). Although some older people can manage today's complex health care system, many more lack the energy, sophistication, cognitive ability, or funds to successfully negotiate a specialty-oriented system. As a result, psychiatrists working with older people must be willing to play a generalist role, combining routine medical management with psychiatric interventions, or helping with specific social or situational problems.

It is also important to have patience and skill in explaining

TABLE 1-3. **Knowledge needed to work effectively with elderly patients**

- Normal aging: biological, psychological, and social changes
- Mental disorders predominantly observed in later life, including dementia of the Alzheimer type, late-onset psychoses
- Effects of age on other psychiatric disorders, including mood and anxiety disorders
- Adjusting psychiatric treatments for aging changes: dose and schedule of psychoactive medications, drug-drug interactions, format and pace of psychotherapy
- Managing social and physical problems of later life: bereavement, role loss, pain, sleep disturbance
- Interactions of psychiatric and medical-surgical illnesses and their treatments

TABLE 1-4. **Personal qualities and professional approaches needed to work effectively with elderly patients**

- Willingness to provide broadly based, flexible management
- Comfortable working closely with other health care professionals
- Patience and skill in providing medical information and assisting in medical decision making
- Willingness to explore one's own feelings about aging
- Openness to discussing patients' concerns about younger professionals
- Acceptance and comfort with limited treatment goals
- Ability to maintain therapeutic optimism in the context of an ultimately poor prognosis

diagnoses and treatments and in assisting older people in medical decision making. Elderly patients often defer to physicians without truly comprehending benefits and risks (17). This may increase efficiency of care in the short run, but may place the older person at risk for iatrogenic illness (e.g., delirium secondary to drug interactions). Finally, it is helpful to have a willingness to explore one's own feelings about aging, as well as being open to discussing older patients' reservations about the wisdom of youth. Elderly patients are inclined to view younger therapists as similar to their children, and therapists, in response, may need to accommodate to relationships involving reverse transference (18).

■ REFERENCES

1. U.S. Senate Special Committee on Aging: Aging America—trends and projections. Washington, DC, U.S. Department of Health and Human Services, 1987–1988
2. Regier DA, Boyd JH, Burke JD, et al: One-month prevalence of mental disorders in the United States. Arch Gen Psychiatry 45:977–986, 1988
3. Rapp SR, Parisi SA, Walsh DA: Psychological dysfunction and physical health among elderly medical inpatients. J Consult Clin Psychol 56:851–855, 1988
4. Small GW, Fawzy FI: Psychiatric consultation for the medically ill elderly in the general hospital: need for a collaborative model of care. Psychosomatics 29:94–103, 1988

5. Rovner BW, Kafonek S, Filipp L, et al: Prevalence of mental illness in a community nursing home. Am J Psychiatry 143:1446–1449, 1986
6. National Institute on Aging Task Force: Senility reconsidered. JAMA 244:259–263, 1980
7. Larson EB, Reifler BV, Sumi SM, et al: Diagnostic evaluation of 200 elderly outpatients with suspected dementia. J Gerontol 40:536–543, 1985
8. Blazer D, Hughes DC, George LK: The epidemiology of depression in an elderly community population. Gerontologist 27:281–287, 1987
9. Gurland GJ, Cross PS: Epidemiology of psychopathology in old age. Psychiatr Clin North Am 5:11–26, 1982
10. Roybal ER: Mental health and aging: the need for an expanded federal response. Am Psychol 43:189–194, 1988
11. U.S. General Accounting Office: The elderly remain in need of mental health services (GAO/HRD-82-112). Washington, DC, U.S. General Accounting Office, 1982
12. Gatz M, Pearson CG: Ageism revised and the provision of psychological services. Am Psychol 43:184–194, 1988
13. Ford CV, Sbordone RJ: Attitudes of psychiatrists toward elderly patients. Am J Psychiatry 137:571–575, 1980
14. Shapiro S, Skinner EA, Kessler LG, et al: Utilization of health and mental health services. Arch Gen Psychiatry 41:971–978, 1984
15. German PS, Shapiro S, Skinner EA, et al: Detection and management of mental health problems of older patients by primary care providers. JAMA 257:489–493, 1987
16. Rapp SR, Davis KM: Geriatric depression: physicians' knowledge, perceptions, and diagnostic practices. Gerontologist 29:242–257, 1989
17. Haug M: Doctor-patient relationships and the older patient. J Gerontol 14:853–860, 1979
18. Berezin MA: Psychodynamic considerations of aging and the aged: an overview. Am J Psychiatry 128:33–41, 1972

■ ADDITIONAL READINGS

Braithwaite VA: Old age stereotypes: reconciling contradictions. J Gerontol 41:353–360, 1986
Kastenbaum R: Personality theory, therapeutic approaches, and the elderly client, in The Clinical Psychology of Aging. Edited by Storandt M, Siegler IC, Elias MF. New York, Plenum, 1978, pp 199–224
Perlick D, Atkins A: Variations in the reported age of a patient: a source of bias in the diagnosis of depression and dementia. J Consult Clin Psychol 52:812–820, 1984

Rowe IW, Grossman E, Bond E, et al: Academic geriatrics for the year 2000: an Institute of Medicine report. N Engl J Med 116:1425–1428, 1987

Small GW, Fong K, Beck JC: Training in geriatric psychiatry: will the supply meet the demand? Am J Psychiatry 145:476–478, 1988

NORMAL AGING 2

■ CONCEPTUAL ISSUES

WHO IS OLD?

In contemporary urban societies, chronological boundaries for life phases such as youth, middle age, and old age are continuously revised upward as medical and social advances extend the vitality and productivity of older adults. The common practice of designating people over the age of 65 as "old" began in Germany in the 1880s, when Otto von Bismarck selected 65 as the starting age for certain social welfare benefits. Whether this should continue to be the qualifying standard, now that so many people live to this point and beyond, is a matter of heated debate among politicians as well as gerontologists.

Psychological and biological aging changes usually occur gradually, without precipitous advances or retreats. To avoid undue emphasis on chronological age, it may be useful to think of each person as having several different ages, e.g., biological, psychological, and social, and to recognize that individuals may be "aged" on one continuum and "youthful" on another (1).

LONGITUDINAL AND CROSS-SECTIONAL VIEWS

The most common way of studying the effects of aging is to compare a group of older people with a separate group of younger adults. Because generational differences are confounded with age when young and old subjects are compared, such cross-sectional investigations often provide an inflated estimate of the magnitude of aging changes.

Longitudinal designs have also been used to study normal aging. These investigations track the same individuals over years, or even decades. The least healthy and able subjects are often the first to drop out from these samples, so unlike cross-sectional studies, longitudinal investigations tend to provide an overly optimistic estimate of the extent of age-related decline.

The best picture of normative aging trends is obtained by combining the results of cross-sectional and longitudinal studies. In Figure 2-1, for example, two curves depict intellectual change with age. The cross-sectional curve, showing progressive decline from mid-life onward, once reflected the predominant view of

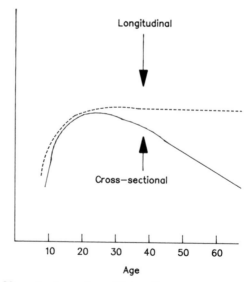

FIGURE 2-1. **Normal aging and cognitive performance—
empirical findings.**

specialists in the field. However, longitudinal data usually show stability in global intellect, at least into early old age. For most aging individuals, reality lies somewhere in between these two views.

HETEROGENEITY IN PATTERNS OF AGING

On many psychological and biological measures, variability is greater in old-age samples than among younger adults. Some of this may be due to the inclusion of medically ill older people in research studies; as a result, ranges of scores reflect effects of illness in addition to age.

Pronounced variability decreases the sensitivity in upper age ranges of many measures that are used to infer pathological change (e.g., clinical electroencephalography, mental status examinations, or depression rating scales). It also casts doubt on the search for singular normative aging trends. In reality, there are probably many different normal aging trajectories, with varying trends for different genetic and sociocultural subgroups. Diversity in aging is difficult to explain at present, but heterogeneity needs to be anticipated, both in research and clinical work.

■ COGNITIVE ABILITIES IN LATER LIFE

Because disorders of cognitive function are so common in later life, it is important to understand the effects of normal aging on cognitive performance. Table 2-1 summarizes age differences in cognitive abilities, and a few of the more important trends are discussed below.

INTELLIGENCE

Intelligence can be thought of as the ability to profit from experience and to adapt to changing life circumstances. In practice, intelligence is usually measured with standardized batteries of tests, such as the Wechsler Adult Intelligence Scales (2).

Studies suggest that some aspects of intelligence remain stable throughout the adult life span, but others routinely decline in later life (3,4). Stable components, often referred to as "crys-

TABLE 2-1. **Age differences in cognitive performance**

Ability	Direction of aging change	Comment
Intelligence		
Crystallized	Stable or increasing	May decline slightly in very old age
Fluid	Declining	Decline begins between ages 55 and 70
Attention		
Attention span	Stable	Digit span unchanged
Complex attention	Declining	Selective or flexible attention declines
Language		
Communication	Stable	In absence of severe sensory deficit
Knowledge of syntax, words	Stable	Influenced by education
Fluency, naming	Declining	Mild problems in lexical access
Comprehension	Stable	Mild decline for complex messages
Discourse	Variable	May be more imprecise, repetitive
Learning and memory		
Sensory memory	Declining	Registration time increased
Immediate memory	Stable	Capacity limited to about 7 ± 2 items
Recent memory	Declining	Encoding, retrieval deficits
Tertiary memory	Variable	Intact for major aspects of personal history
Visuospatial ability		
Design copying	Variable	Intact for simple figures; errors on 3-dimensional designs
Topographic orientation	Declining	Especially in unfamiliar places

TABLE 2-1. Age differences in cognitive performance
(continued)

Ability	Direction of aging change	Comment
Reasoning ability		
Logical problem solving	Declining	Mild problems with redundancy, disorganization
Practical reasoning	Variable	May differ for novel, familiar tasks

tallized" intelligence, include the ability to define and use words (vocabulary), to access general cultural knowledge (information), and to engage in practical and social reasoning (comprehension). By contrast, performance of novel, speeded, perceptual-motor tasks, which tap "fluid" intellectual abilities, generally diminishes with age. Examples of these tasks include arranging blocks to form specific patterns (block design), ordering pictures so that they tell a meaningful story (picture arrangement), or identifying missing parts of pictures (picture completion).

Crystallized intelligence is maintained through education and accumulated cultural experience, whereas fluid intellectual abilities are thought to reflect neurobiological function (4). Precise brain-behavior relationships have not been identified. One neuropsychological hypothesis stresses the similarity between performance in older adults and in patients with right hemisphere brain lesions; however, most evidence suggests that brain changes occur bilaterally in normal aging. Another neuropsychological model compares older adults with patients with frontal or subcortical brain lesions (5). There are some neurobiological findings consistent with this idea (e.g., decreased numbers of large neurons in the frontal cortex and scattered reports of hypometabolism of glucose in selected frontal regions). However, the intellectual changes observed with normal aging are equally consistent with a hypothesis of mild, diffuse brain changes.

Fluid intellectual declines might be considered an artifact of behavioral slowing. Reduced performance speed is probably the most reliable behavior change associated with advancing age.

Some reduction results from peripheral factors, such as decreased speed of nerve conduction or diminished muscle mass. However, central decision-making speed also declines with age, most noticeably on complex or difficult tasks. Therefore, older adults' mental slowing is best viewed as an integral part of intellectual decline, much as it is in neuropsychological assessment of younger brain-injured patients.

LEARNING AND MEMORY

When older people complain about their cognitive abilities, they usually mention problems with memory. Research substantiates these complaints, but also indicates that some aspects of memory decline more with age than others (6).

Short-term, or immediate, memory does not change appreciably with age. For example, older people do about as well as young adults on digit- or word-span tests that require retention of small amounts of information for short periods of time.

Anecdotally, remote or long-term memory is also well maintained in old age. Research results are not so clear, partly because remote memory is hard to measure because initial or intervening exposure to the material cannot be precisely controlled. Overall, however, older adults' absolute levels of performance on remote-memory tests are often impressively high; for example, one study found that people recognized names or photos of more than 70% of their high school classmates after an interval of almost 50 years.

The largest age decrements are observed in recent, or secondary, memory. Age differences favoring the young have been found on many different tests of recent memory, such as remembering items on shopping lists, learning to associate pairs of words, copying designs from memory, or remembering content of stories and conversations. Normal elderly people even make more mistakes than young adults on memory items from mental status examinations, such as 5-minute delayed recall of three or four simple words.

Some of the decline in recent memory has been traced to problems with initial learning (3,6). Many older people take a more passive approach to learning and remembering than younger adults. For example, elderly people report less spontaneous use of mnemonic strategies than younger people and do not appear to capitalize as readily on the organization inherent in words or actions as a basis for learning and recall. However, if explicitly instructed to use mnemonics or organizational strategies, older individuals' performance often improves dramatically, at least in the short run. Long-term evaluations of memory-training programs have produced discouraging results, because most older people stop using mnemonic strategies within a few weeks or months of training.

Active encoding and retrieval may require greater expenditure of effort and energy than most older people can afford. Declines in effortful processing may be due to altered neurotransmitter functions (especially catecholamines). Alternatively, such processing changes may be seen as an adaptive response to the diminished demands of older adults' everyday life-styles. Also, it is important to note that there are some very healthy and active elderly people who do as well on demanding memory tasks as more average young adults.

REASONING AND DECISION MAKING

Most older people feel that their problem-solving abilities improve with age. However, research does not agree with this self-appraisal. Elderly adults identify concepts more slowly than young adults and are often less organized in asking questions or evaluating different solutions to problems (3). As complexity of problems increases, they may be prone to "overload" and fail to make reasonable choices.

Older people may find it easier to solve real-life problems than abstract research tasks (3). However, medical decision making is an area where the elderly usually feel ineffectual, and the limited research available bears out their difficulties in comprehending informed consent procedures (7). Simplifying language and providing pictures or examples may be necessary to make complex medical information clear to older patients.

CLINICAL IMPLICATIONS OF COGNITIVE CHANGE

The prevalence of cognitive declines in normal aging increases the risk of diagnostic errors, particularly overdiagnosis of organic mental disorders. On the Mini-Mental State Exam, for example, one study found that 21% of subjects over age 60 scored below the typical cutoff for cognitive impairment (i.e., 23 or fewer correct out of 30) (8). Five percent had only 17 or fewer correct, and of these, a substantial subgroup (14%) were found to be without diagnosable mental disorder on detailed psychiatric and neuro-logic examination. Therefore, when using a cognitive mental status examination with older people, it is important to interpret outcomes cautiously and to follow up with more thorough diagnostic assessment for those who score in the impaired range. Paying attention to the pattern and types of errors may also help to distinguish normal from abnormal cognitive changes. Table 2-2 summarizes some hallmarks of normal older adults' performance on mental status examinations.

TABLE 2-2. **Performance of older adults on mental status examinations**

Within normal limits	Raises question of impairment
Orientation	
Well oriented to place and time	Errors on $\geq$75% of questions
May miss specific date, address	Far-miss responses (e.g., 1978 for 1989)
Registration	
Can easily repeat 3 or 4 words	Paraphasias or omissions
Attention	
Can repeat 5–7 digits	Forward digit span < 5
Can count backward from 20 or recite alphabet quickly, with no errors	Errors on simple mental-control tests
Understands serial 7s, but may make subtraction errors	Cannot comprehend task, gross errors (e.g., adding or counting)

TABLE 2-2. **Performance of older adults on mental status examinations** *(continued)*

Within normal limits	Raises question of impairment
Delayed recall	
May miss 1 or 2 out of 3 or 4 items	Confabulation, intrusion errors
Can remember missed items when given cues or multiple choices	Failure to benefit from cues or multiple choices
Language	
Can quickly name common objects	Paraphasias
Can name at least 10 words in a common category in 1 minute; expect more if well educated	Perseverations, intrusions
Can read and write sentences in primary language	Nonsensical responses, perseveration
Design copying	
Accurate copies of 2-dimensional figures	Problems with 2-dimensional figures
Mild errors in detail on 3-dimensional designs	Gross distortions, perseverations, rotations
Abstraction	
Depends on education: abstract if well educated, may be concrete on similarities or proverbs with little formal education	Bizarre associations, interpretations
Everyday judgment intact	Impulsivity, disorganized responses

Age-related cognitive changes also have implications for the doctor-patient relationship and for selection and monitoring of treatment. As previously noted, extra care may be required in explaining medical procedures to ensure informed decision making. In psychotherapy, the reduced pace of new learning and changes in reasoning processes may result in a slower rate of clinical improvement. Often, this can be dealt with effectively by increasing the number of therapy sessions.

Abrupt changes in cognitive function always warrant medical attention. Even more gradual declines, emerging over a year or two, may be an early warning of occult illness (so-called terminal decline) and should be carefully monitored (see Table 2-3).

■ PERSONALITY AND EMOTIONAL CHANGES

Personality has not been as thoroughly studied as cognition in old age. However, available data suggest that there may be important normative trends in this area of behavior as well.

COEXISTING STABILITY AND CHANGE

Many basic personality dispositions develop early in life and persist throughout adult years, but there is also evidence for change in adult personality. One study traced the relative prominence of different personal qualities (e.g., assertiveness, cheerful-

TABLE 2-3. **Indications of possible "terminal decline"**

Based on consecutive evaluations across a period of 1 or 2 years:

- Any drop in vocabulary ability
  Rationale: This ability is very stable, and may even increase, in normal old age.
- Decline in verbal abstraction (e.g., >10% loss on Wechsler Adult Intelligence Scale—Revised (WAIS-R) similarities score per year)
  Rationale: As a group, older adults are often more concrete than younger people, but this may be due to education or other cultural differences. Intraindividual change in verbal abstraction is negligible.
- Decline in speeded, perceptual-motor ability (e.g., >2% loss in WAIS-R digit symbol score per year)
  Rationale: Some reduction in speed and perceptual-motor ability is expected with normal aging. However, this change occurs slowly and would not normally be clinically noticeable over a 1- to 2-year period.

Note. These trends may not be applicable for very old individuals (80+ years).
Source. Adapted from Jarvik LF, Bank L: Aging twins: longitudinal psychometric data, in Longitudinal Studies of Adult Development. Edited by Schaie KW. New York, Guilford, 1983, pp 40–63.

ness, hostility) from early adolescence to mid-life and early old age (9). Most qualities retained their original degree of importance in people's makeups, including basic tempo or activity level, styles of cognitive engagement, modes of self-presentation, and pathological tendencies. However, other characteristics underwent "ordered transition," shifting upward or downward in a consistent way with increasing age. These orderly changes were more common among women than men and included such shifts as increasing aspiration levels and declining reliance on conventionality. In addition, there were some aspects of personality that changed erratically over the years, increasing at one point, then fading in prominence at others.

INFLUENCES ON ADULT PERSONALITY

Precise patterns of ebb and flow in personality probably vary with generations, because each cohort encounters a unique set of pressures and opportunities at successive life phases. However, certain causal processes appear to be consistently important. One influential developmental force is the "social clock" (10). Most societies have rather firm beliefs about age appropriateness of various actions. Some of these beliefs are formalized through minimum age laws or standards (e.g., for marriage, voting, or retirement), but most are informally imposed. The social clock sets the pace for psychosocial development within a given generation and provides a standard that individuals may internalize as a normal, expectable life cycle.

A second important force is the individual's desire for continuity in personal past and present. Continuity has been described as "a grand adaptive strategy" promoted by individual preference and reinforced by social approval (11). The search for continuity may be at the heart of reminiscence, which occurs at all ages, and of the process of life review that is so common among elderly adults.

Individual and social influences may combine to produce ordered transitions or stages in adult personality. Erikson's (12) widely cited theory depicts development as progressing through eight age-correlated phases. Each stage is associated with a primary developmental task, and accomplishment of each task has a bearing on subsequent stages. In late adulthood, the primary task concerns integrity versus despair; i.e., each person is faced with making sense of his or her actions over a lifetime, and with judging the purpose and impact of these behaviors. Morale in old age may depend on success in resolving this issue, in addition to those of earlier life phases.

STRESS AND COPING IN OLD AGE

Specific losses that accompany old age (e.g., bereavement, disability, retirement) can also affect morale and subjective well-being. The elderly may be particularly vulnerable to such losses because of negative age stereotypes, which may be internalized at times of high stress (see Figure 2-2). In this view, emotional problems in old age result from a cyclic process set in motion by societal biases and the loss of social roles, rather than from disruptions of intrapsychic development.

Older people tend to cope with stressful events in different ways than younger adults, relying more often on emotion-focused forms of coping, as opposed to active, problem-solving approaches (13). Emotion-based coping is more passive than confrontational, more individual than interpersonal, and oriented toward control of distressing feelings rather than altering stressful situations. Examples of emotion-focused coping include distancing from the problem, accepting responsibility, and positive reappraisal. The elderly also tend to see their situations as less changeable than younger adults, and to the extent that this is true, their preferred forms of coping may be highly adaptive. However, more direct forms of problem solving may need to be encouraged in specific cases.

Locus of control is another dimension that affects response to stressful situations. For example, older people who believe that their health is controlled by powerful others adjust better to acute-care hospitals and high-constraint long-term care than those who see their physical well-being as under their own control. In the community, belief in external locus of control is associated with increased visits to physicians during times of very high stress. However, regardless of preexisting control orientation, studies of long-term care show that sense of well-being tends to increase when residents are given greater opportunities to regulate their own environment (14).

Although old age presents many personal and social obstacles, poor morale has been found to be the exception rather than the rule among older adults. In one recent poll of relatively healthy people, 60% of respondents 50 and older said they were "very satisfied" with their lives, compared to 53% of those between the ages of 18 and 49 (15). Most respondents over age 50 said that theirs was the "ideal age," whereas people between 18 and 49 generally thought the best age to be 29 or younger.

CLINICAL IMPLICATIONS OF PERSONALITY DEVELOPMENT

Core features of personality remain stable throughout adulthood, and any marked change in mood or social behavior should raise a question of pathology. However, more subtle reordering of personal priorities and shifts in coping styles are not inconsistent with normal aging. It is particularly important not to measure older people's coping by youthful standards. Emotion-focused coping may be a sign of wisdom rather than regression, particularly if the

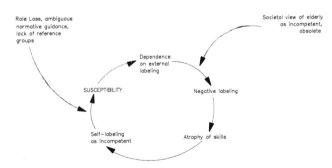

FIGURE 2-2. **Social breakdown cycle in old age.** Adapted with permission from Kuypers JA, Bengtson VL: Social breakdown and competence: a model of normal aging. Human Development 16:190, 1973. Copyright 1973 S. Karger AG, Basel.

problem being faced (e.g., bereavement or serious illness) is hard to resolve through action.

In acute-care situations, it is important to accurately appraise an individual's beliefs about locus of control. Those with internal locus of control adjust best if given a chance to participate in medical decision making, whereas those who believe in external control may benefit more from knowing that they are attended by recognized experts. Those who suspect that their fate depends on chance may adjust best if the care environment is consistent and predictable.

Older people can benefit from the full range of psychotherapies used with younger people. There are some highly educated and thoughtful elderly people who are well suited for long-term therapy addressing intrapsychic tasks of later life. For many others, situational interventions, aimed at modifying real-life problems, may be most appropriate. In either case, goal setting for the future should be part of the psychotherapy agenda.

■ THE SOCIAL CONTEXT OF AGING

Old age is accompanied by role change and, often, role loss. Most people can expect transformations in occupational, family, and community roles, and for many, the number of different roles declines in later life.

WORK AND FINANCIAL STATUS

Most elderly adults are retired from full-time work. In 1986, only 25% of men aged 65–69 were working for pay, and among those aged 70 and above, only 10% were employed (16). Participation of older people in the labor force has declined sharply over recent decades, primarily because of improvements in pension plans. However, a growing number have part-time, paid employment and about one in five are active as volunteers. Although people report that they miss the money and opportunities for social contact that everyday work provides, most take retirement in stride, adopting new routines and activities to take the place of work. This is particularly likely when retirement is predictable or self-imposed, and when postretirement income is adequate.

Health problems, either physical or mental, usually do not increase in the weeks or months after retirement. However, retirement that occurs much earlier or later than the norm (i.e., at or about age 65) may be associated with greater symptoms of mental distress.

Because of Social Security and other pension programs, a majority of older people are financially independent of younger relatives. Social Security provides about 37% of total income for Americans 65 and older. An additional 13% comes from other pension funds, 23% from investment income, and 25% from current earnings. Less than 2% is directly provided by children.

MARRIAGE AND WIDOWHOOD

Marital relationships in old age differ sharply for women and men. About 50% of women 65 and older are widows, and another 11% are single, divorced, or living apart from their spouses (16). For women 75 and older, two in three are widowed and less than 25% are married and living with their husbands. By contrast, 75% of men aged 65 or older and 68% of those 75 and older are living with their wives (16).

Bereavement results in increased depressive symptoms and a decline in positive affect (see Chapter 3). Usually, these problems resolve within a year or two of a spouse's death. Also, normal bereavement generally does not produce a loss of self-esteem or inappropriate guilt. However, men, and women with few friends, tend to have a harder time adjusting to widowhood. For those with long-term marriages that continue into old age, satisfaction may increase in later life compared with earlier marital phases.

CHILDREN, SIBLINGS, AND FRIENDS

Compared with younger people, the elderly tend to have smaller social networks and less frequent interpersonal contacts (17). Older people also rely more heavily on family members and long-term friendships for input on important matters. Nearly 80% of older adults have at least one living child, and at least two-thirds report that they have seen their children within the past week; others maintain frequent contact by telephone (16). Contact with children is a valued source of emotional gratification for most older people, including the very old.

The elderly are also actively involved with their siblings. As individuals recognize themselves as aging, sibling relationships appear to increase in importance, with sisters playing a particularly active role in maintaining kinship networks.

Intimate, confiding relationships may be most valuable to people's well-being and mental health in old age. About four out of five elderly people report having confidants, and many have several. When available, spouses are most likely to be listed as confidants, followed by friends, children, and siblings.

ASSISTANCE ACROSS GENERATIONS

One of the most prominent fears of elderly people is the specter of becoming a burden on their children (16). Research substantiates that the elderly receive much assistance from their children, but the reverse is also true. In one national survey, more than one-half of the respondents 65 and older were helping younger family members, taking care of relatives when ill, baby-sitting grandchildren, providing loans or gifts of money, and offering advice with life's problems. Assistance from children is more readily accepted by those who are satisfied with the contributions that they have made to their children's welfare in the past. In general, however, children are more willing to give assistance than older people are to receive it. It may be helpful to encourage conflicted older people to view assistance from younger relatives as withdrawal from a "support bank" (18) to which they have contributed throughout their lives.

IMPLICATIONS OF SOCIAL CONTEXT FOR CLINICAL CARE

Psychiatrists need to identify sources of social support for older people, facilitate meaningful contacts for those without social networks, and promote reciprocity in assistance where possible. Intergenerational family therapy can be useful, particularly if it reinforces older patients' ability to give as well as to receive.

Because older women are frequently widowed and may outlive other kin, they are especially likely to find themselves alone in advanced old age. Women may be more adept than men at forming friendships in later life, but this possible strength may be counteracted by physical or sensory disability. For those with very restricted social resources, therapists must sometimes be willing to provide periodic support on a long-term basis.

■ BIOLOGICAL AGING

THEORIES OF AGING

A useful definition of aging was proposed by Birren and Zarit (19): "Biological aging, senescing, is the process of change in the organism, which over time lowers the probability of survival and reduces the physiological capacity for self-regulation, repair and adaptation to environmental demands" (p. 9). Modern gerontologists distinguish primary aging, which is postulated to reflect an intrinsic, presumably genetically preprogrammed limit on cellular longevity, from secondary aging, which is due to the accumulated effects of environmental insult, disease, and trauma. Primary aging seems to account for the relatively constant maximum life span observed in almost all animal species studied, whereas secondary aging explains much of the variability among individual members of a species.

That primary aging is "built into" the cell was first appreciated by Hayflick and associates (20,21) in a series of experiments that established the maximum number of cell divisions ("doublings") that would take place in carefully cultured normal human cells at about 50, plus or minus 10. As cultured cells approach this limit, losses in many functional capacities are observed, with the final cessation of cellular reproduction apparently reflecting accumulated functional losses. Evidence that the "Hayflick phenomenon" is under genetic control includes *1*) a fair correlation between the doubling limit and the maximum species-specific life span of the cell donor, and *2*) a reduced doubling limit in cells cultured from patients with genetic diseases of accelerated aging, such as progeria (Hutchinson-Gilford syndrome) and Werner's syndrome. The observation that cells in culture retain their preprogrammed doubling limit even after being frozen for years suggests that the doubling limit is not related only to total time elapsed, whereas the observed inverse relationship between doubling capacity and the age of the cell donor indicates that the limit is not just an in vitro phenomenon; that is, doublings in vivo appear to "count" as well as those that occur in vitro. Similar losses of functional capacity (i.e., cellular aging) have since been observed in all cell types studied, including those with little or no reproductive capacity, such as neurons.

The precise mechanism whereby genes enforce this limit remains unknown. Many contemporary theories of aging entail the notion of accumulated error. According to these theories, processes involved in cellular metabolism (for example, protein synthesis) are imperfect, and small errors occur now and then. Over time, the consequences of these small errors add up to cellular aging and death. Other accumulation theories identify environmentally induced mutations in the genome, or the deleterious auto-oxidizing effects of "free radicals," or the development of cross-linkages in collagen as the fundamental cause of tissue aging. It is possible that genetic mechanisms at least partially determine vulnerability to accumulated error and insult, much in the way that some types of automobiles, on the basis of their design, outlast and require less repair than others. Although there is evidence in support of each of these theories, a comprehensive theory of aging that captures most of the observed facts of primary biological aging remains to be articulated.

PRIMARY AGING: STRUCTURAL AND FUNCTIONAL CHANGES

The major structural changes in humans that have been attributed to primary aging are listed, by organ system, in Table 2-4, along with the major functional consequences of these changes. Be cautioned that cross-sectional studies produced most of the tabulated findings. In addition to the general shortcomings of such studies described above, data on the anatomical and physiological effects of age are usually confounded by selection bias (i.e., rarely are "random samples" studied in this type of research) as well as the uncontrollable effects of "secondary" aging.

TABLE 2-4. **Primary aging changes in anatomy and function of major organ systems**

System	Anatomical	Functional
Cardiovascular		
Heart	Decreased size. Lipofuscin and fat deposition in myocardium; loss of flexibility of collagen matrix. Fatty infiltration and calcification of aortic and mitral valves.	Resting data conflict: One study showed about 1% per year reduction of cardiac index between the ages of 20 and 80; another showed no changes over the same age range. Under stress: reduced maximal heart rate, stroke volume, cardiac output, and oxygen consumption.
Arteries	Redistribution and molecular rearrangement of elastin in arterial walls; calcification.	Loss of elasticity, increased systolic blood pressure.
Respiratory		
Lungs	Enlargement of aveolar ducts and alveoli, loss of elasticity.	Reduced ventilatory capacity, especially during exercise.
Musculoskeletal	Increased chest wall and joint rigidity, increased kyphosis, calcification of cartilage.	Reduced ventilatory capacity, especially during exercise.
Gastrointestinal	Some loss of smooth muscle cells of intestine, atrophy of gastric mucosa, and increased gastric pH. Some loss of hepatocytes and reduction of hepatic blood flow.	Reduced eliminatory efficiency: constipation. Reduced metabolism of drugs (see below).
Genitourinary	Loss of renal mass, including loss of glomeruli. Reduced intrarenal arterial tree. Reduced bladder elasticity, especially in females. Prostate enlargement in males.	Reduced glomerular filtration rate and renal plasma flow. Loss of bladder emptying capacity.

TABLE 2-4. **Primary aging changes in anatomy and function of major organ systems** *(continued)*

System	Anatomical	Functional
Endocrinologic	Atrophy and fibrosis, loss of vascularity. Changes may be very minimal.	General decline in secretory rate, but resting hormone blood levels may remain constant as clearance also declines.
Nervous	Loss of brain weight and volume in most studies. Loss of neurons, depending on brain area studied. Loss of dendritic arbor of neurons, with reduced interneuronal connectivity. Interneuronal accumulation of lipofuscin and loss of organelles. Neurofibrillary degeneration of neurons, and accumulation of senile plaques, especially in hippocampus, amygdala, and frontal cortex.	Inconsistent findings, with some investigators reporting reduced cerebral blood flow, reduced metabolism of glucose and oxygen, others failing to find these changes. Intellectual changes as described above.
Musculoskeletal	Reduced muscle, bone mass. Increased fat in muscles, calcium in cartilage. Loss of elasticity in joints.	Loss of muscular strength and stamina.
Immunologic	Increased T suppressor, decreased helper T cells. Increased IgA and IgG, decreased IgM. Increased autoantibodies. Involution of thymus gland.	Increased susceptibility to infection, cancer.
Special senses	Yellowing of lens.	Loss of auditory and visual acuity, especially night vision.

■ IMPLICATIONS OF BIOLOGICAL AGING FOR PSYCHIATRIC TREATMENT

PSYCHOSOCIAL THERAPIES

Older patients may require that the therapist modify his or her technique in order to optimally benefit from psychotherapy. Sensory losses may require that the therapist sit closer and speak louder and more slowly than would be appropriate for middle-aged patients. Amplification devices may be of value; generally desk-top systems offer much greater clarity and resolution than standard hearing aids. Impaired short-term memory may require that the therapist reiterate key points several times and may contribute to learning difficulties that are indistinguishable from resistance and denial. For example, older patients may be more prone to forget appointments and may need reminder calls. Sensory losses and reduced short-term memory may contribute to a generalized reduction in attention span and decreased capacity for therapeutic work, so sessions may need to be shorter than with younger patients. Musculoskeletal aging may impair mobility and interfere with patients' ability to get to appointments, and the role of telephone contact in their care may be expanded.

PSYCHOPHARMACOLOGIC THERAPIES

PHARMACOKINETICS

Of the four major determinants of pharmacokinetics—absorption, distribution, metabolism, and excretion—all but absorption are significantly affected by normal aging changes.

The majority of studies indicate that the rate of gastrointestinal absorption of most drugs is essentially unimpaired by the atrophy of gastric mucosa, increased pH, and reduced splanchnic blood flow associated with aging (22,23).

The distribution of drugs in the body, on the other hand, is more reliably altered by the aging process, primarily as a result of relative loss of body water and lean body mass. Both of these changes result in relatively increased plasma concentrations of drugs that are distributed in body water, such as lithium carbonate, or in lean body mass, such as digoxin (24). Conversely, drugs that deposit in lean body mass and adipose tissue, such as diazepam, are distributed in a larger "apparent volume" (25) and will attain somewhat lower plasma concentrations than in a younger patient.

Aging is also associated with reduced amounts (in the range of a 20% reduction) of serum albumin, the serum protein most highly "bound" to drugs in plasma. For drugs that are highly (i.e., over 95%) albumin bound, such as furosemide or warfarin, this reduction may "free" a significantly higher proportion of drug for distribution to its site of action, with resultant greater drug effect.

After distribution, most drugs undergo two-phase metabolism in the liver. The first phase is oxidation, reduction, or hydrolysis; these reactions are catalyzed by enzymes in the microsomal fraction of homogenated liver tissue. The second phase of metabolism is acetylation, or conjugation with glucuronide, sulfate, or glycine; second-phase metabolism usually produces active or inactive water-soluble compounds that are then excreted by the kidney. Although reductions in hepatic blood flow (about 45% between the ages of 25 and 65), relative hepatic mass (about one-third), and hepatic enzyme activity have been demonstrated in elderly individuals, examination of the actual rate of metabolism of drugs in elderly subjects has produced contradictory results, and few generalizations are possible. One such generalization is that hepatic conjugation of drugs is relatively spared by age effects; the significance of this sparing with respect to benzodiazepine therapy is clear in Table 2-5.

Age effects on renal excretion of drugs have been much more clearly delineated. Reduction of glomerular filtration (which generally corresponds to rate of excretion of drugs) of approximately 1% per year between the ages of 30 and 80 has been documented, as has comparable reduction in renal plasma flow and renal tubular function, including absorption and secretion (26). For drugs that are excreted by the kidney unchanged, like lithium salts, or that have active water-soluble metabolites, like desipramine (i.e., 2-OH-desipramine), this reduction may have great clinical significance. For other agents whose water-soluble metabolites are inactive, this change is less important.

TABLE 2-5. **Age-related change in elimination half-life (T½) of selected benzodiazepines**

Agent	Change in T½
Oxazepam	No change
Lorazepam	No change
Alprazolam	Approx. 50% increase, M > F
Diazepam	Approx. 100% increase, M > F
Chlordiazepoxide	Approx. 100% increase, M > F

Note. M = male. F = female.

PHARMACODYNAMICS

Pharmacodynamics refers to the actual physiological response produced by a drug at its site of action. When pharmacokinetic factors are constant, increased or decreased effectiveness of drugs can be assumed to reflect pharmacodynamic changes. Only a few such changes have been documented in normal elderly patients: increased sensitivity to the central nervous system depressant effects of benzodiazepine anxiolytics and hypnotics (27), increased sensitivity to the effects of warfarin, and decreased sensitivity to the chronotropic effects of isoproterenol.

PRESCRIBING PSYCHOACTIVE MEDICATIONS

The implication of age-related changes in the pharmacokinetics and pharmacodynamics of psychoactive medications can be stated in a few simple rules of thumb:

- Determine the patient's baseline physiologic status before initiating therapy; this usually requires evaluation of hepatic and renal function and the function of any organ or organ system that may be adversely affected by medications, e.g., an electrocardiogram should be obtained before initiating therapy with tricyclic antidepressants.
- Start with relatively small doses, for example, one-third to one-half of the normal "adult" dose.

- If dosage increase is indicated, proceed slowly.
- Be particularly alert for the development of adverse reactions and side effects.

Some do's and don'ts for geriatric psychopharmacology:

- *Do identify appropriate target symptoms.* Failure to do so is a common cause of treatment failure. Target symptoms may be absolutely inappropriate, e.g., social withdrawal in a depressed patient who is characterologically antisocial, unhappiness and dissatisfaction in a patient who feels stuck in a bad marriage, etc., or temporally inappropriate. An example of the latter is adjusting antipsychotic therapy to elimination of delusional content while failing to appreciate improved behavior and reduced agitation; the latter are appropriate early indicators of adequate treatment, whereas the former may require months of therapy. Similarly, typical early indicators of response to antidepressants are improvement in sleep, appetite, and anxiety; subjective improvement in mood usually appears later in the course of therapy. In general, global improvement is an undesirable target of therapy, as it is relatively more sensitive to vicissitudes of daily life, subject to more interrater variability, and more influenceable by the mood and expectations of a single rater than are more concrete targets such as appetite or sleep, or specific psychological states like hopelessness, helplessness, and anhedonia.
- *Do change one thing at a time.* One goal of psychopharmacotherapy is to identify ineffective approaches. Only if treatment is conducted systematically, adequate dosages are prescribed, adequate amounts of time are allowed, and changes are made one at a time is it possible to learn which treatments are ineffective or unnecessary and need no further exploration. For example, a patient is unresponsive to a tricyclic antidepressant, so the dose is increased and lithium is added, and rapid response follows. Which maneuver is responsible? Is the lithium necessary? Would a higher dose alone have sufficed?
- *Don't use medications for their side effects.* Common violations of this principle include prescribing increasing amounts of neuroleptic medications when sedation is desired, prescribing antihistamines for their hypnotic or anticholinergic side effects, or prescribing antidepressants as hypnotics for

nondepressed patients. Failure to follow this principle with elderly patients increases the risk of adverse reactions due to overtreatment, e.g., neuroleptic malignant syndrome or anticholinergic delirium. This principle does not discourage selection of an agent when its therapeutic effects and its side effects are both desirable, such as the selection of a sedating antidepressant for a depressed patient with sleep disturbance.

- *Do maintain an optimistic and supportive attitude.* This is particularly important during the first few days and weeks of therapy when the ratio of side effects to clinical gain is particularly low. Optimism does not entail or justify unrealistic expectations, but helps to maximize the placebo effect, which has been shown to account for about one-half of the efficacy of psychopharmacologic agents.

- *Don't undertreat.* The geriatric literature appropriately emphasizes the hazards of overtreatment and unnecessary polypharmacy. However, because of the increased sensitivity of most elderly patients to medication side effects, the clinician usually has clear signals indicating overtreatment. Such is not the case with undertreatment, where partial response can "freeze" therapy at a suboptimal level. Often it is diagnostic uncertainty or therapeutic timidity on the part of the clinician that leads to these outcomes. A good rule of thumb is to increase dosages until clear clinical response has occurred; if response diminishes or plateaus short of complete remission, dosages should be increased again, with the ceiling defined as development of minor side effects that do not remit over several days. At this point, minor dosage reduction may be appropriate. In this way, the clinician can be reasonably confident that the most effective (i.e., the highest) dosage possible for that patient has been reached. Of course, with certain agents such as nortriptyline, where a true "therapeutic window" may exist, this approach requires particularly close monitoring of clinical response and determination of serum drug levels.

■ REFERENCES

1. Birren JE, Cunningham W: Research on the psychology of aging: principles, concepts, and theory, in Handbook of the Psychology of

Aging, 2nd Edition. Edited by Birren JE, Schaie KW. New York, Van Nostrand Reinhold, 1985, pp 3–34

2. Wechsler D: Wechsler Adult Intelligence Scale—Revised. New York, Psychological Corporation, 1981

3. Botwinick J: Aging and Behavior, 3rd Edition. New York, Springer, 1984

4. Horn JL: The aging of human abilities, in Handbook of Developmental Psychology. Edited by Wolman BB. Englewood Cliffs, NJ, Prentice-Hall, 1982, pp 267–300

5. Hochanadel G, Kaplan E: Neuropsychology of normal aging, in Clinical Neurology of Aging. Edited by Albert ML. New York, Oxford University Press, 1984, pp 231–244

6. Kaszniak AW, Poon LW, Riege W: Assessing memory deficits: an information-processing approach, in Handbook for Clinical Memory Assessment of Older Adults. Edited by Poon L. Washington, DC, American Psychological Association, 1986, pp 168–188

7. Tymchuk AJ, Ouslander JG, Rader N: Informing the elderly: a comparison of four methods. J Am Geriatr Soc 34:818–822, 1986

8. Folstein MF, Anthony JC, Parhad I, et al: The meaning of cognitive impairment in the elderly. J Am Geriatr Soc 33:228–235, 1985

9. Haan H, Day D: A longitudinal study of change and sameness in personality development: adolescence to later adulthood. Int J Aging Hum Dev 5:11–39, 1974

10. Neugarten BL: Adaptation and the life cycle. J Geriatr Psychiatry 4:71–85, 1970

11. Atchley RC: A continuity theory of normal aging. Gerontologist 29:183–190, 1989

12. Erikson E: Childhood and Society. New York, WW Norton, 1950

13. Folkman S, Lazarus RS, Pimley S, et al: Age differences in stress and coping processes. Psychology and Aging 2:171–184, 1987

14. Langer EJ, Rodin J: The effects of choice and enhanced personal responsibility for the aged. J Pers Soc Psychol 34:191–198, 1976

15. Roark AC: Most older persons say they're happy with lives. Los Angeles Times, May 4, 1989, pp 1, 24–25

16. U.S. Senate Special Committee on Aging: Aging America—trends and projections. Washington, DC, U.S. Department of Health and Human Services, 1987–1988

17. Morgan D: Age differences in social network participation. J Gerontol 43:S129–S137, 1988

18. Antonucci T: Personal characteristics, social support, and social behavior, in Handbook of Aging and the Social Sciences. Edited by Binstock T, Shanas E. New York, Van Nostrand Reinhold, 1985, pp 94–128

19. Birren JE, Zarit J: Concepts of health, behavior, and aging, in Cognition, Stress and Aging. Edited by Birren JE, Livingston J. Englewood Cliffs, NJ, Prentice-Hall, 1985, pp 1–18
20. Hayflick L, Moorhead PS: The serial cultivation of human diploid cell strains. Exp Cell Res 25:585–621, 1961
21. Hayflick L: The limited in vitro lifetime of human diploid cell strains. Exp Cell Res 37:614–636, 1965
22. Shader RI, Greenblatt DJ, Ciraulo DA, et al: Effect of age and sex on disposition of desmethyldiazepam formed from its precursor clorazepate. Psychopharmacology 75:193–197, 1981
23. Greenblatt DJ, Divoll M, Harmatz JS, et al: Oxazepam kinetics: effects of age and sex. J Pharmacol Exp Ther 215:86–91, 1980
24. Cusak B, Kelly J, O'Malley K, et al: Digoxin in the elderly: pharmacokinetic consequences of old age. Clin Pharmacol Ther 25:772–776, 1979
25. Greenblatt DJ, Allen MD, Harmatz JS, et al: Diazepam disposition determinants. Clin Pharmacol Ther 27:301–312, 1980
26. Rowe JW, Andres R, Tobin JD, et al: The effect of age on creatinine clearance in man. J Gerontol 31:155–163, 1976
27. Greenblatt DJ, Allen MD, Shader RI: Toxicity of high-dose flurazepam in the elderly. Clin Pharmacol Ther 21:355–361, 1977

■ ADDITIONAL READINGS

Butler RN: Successful aging and the role of the life review. J Am Geriatr Soc 22:529–535, 1974
Carstensen LL, Edelstein BA (eds): Handbook of Clinical Gerontology (General Psychology Series). Elmsford, NY, 1987
Cicirelli VC: Locus of control and patient role adjustment of the elderly in acute-care hospitals. Psychology and Aging 2:138–143, 1987
Finch CE, Schneider EL (eds): Handbook of the Biology of Aging, 2nd Edition. New York, Van Nostrand Reinhold, 1985
Gould RL: Transformations: Growth and Change in Adult Life. New York, Simon & Schuster, 1978
Litwak E: Helping Older People: The Complementary Roles of Informal Networks and Formal Systems. New York, Guilford, 1985

3 MOOD DISORDERS—DIAGNOSIS

■ MAJOR DEPRESSION

Major depression is the most serious presentation of mood disorder in the elderly. It occurs in about 1–4% of individuals over age 65 (1,2) and accounts for over 60% of admissions to geriatric psychiatry units (3); depression accounts for almost one-half of admissions of elderly persons to psychiatric hospitals in general (4) and is present in about 30% of elderly patients with acute and chronic medical illness (5).

Major depression affects the elderly in many of the same ways it does young adults. However, the relative prominence of certain diagnostic features has been found to vary with age. Older depressed patients less commonly complain of diminished self-esteem and guilt, whereas somatic complaints, difficulty concentrating, memory impairment, and reduced energy are seen more commonly in the elderly. In addition, because several features of normal aging overlap with complaints of depression, accurate detection of major depression in old age can be challenging. Table 3-1 lists the most troublesome of these normal aging changes. In addition to normal aging changes, changes associated with normal bereavement may further complicate diagnosis and must be ruled out before major depression can be diagnosed. Finally, as discussed below, accurate diagnosis of major depression may also be complicated by variable presentation of illness.

VARIATIONS IN CLINICAL PRESENTATION

PSYCHOTIC DEPRESSION

Of several clinical variants common in elderly patients, perhaps the most frequently seen is psychotic depression, reported to occur in over 40% of admissions to a psychogeriatric inpatient service (6). Identification of this syndrome as a mood disorder is relatively straightforward when symptoms occur in the "classical" sequence, i.e., when mood and neurovegetative changes occur before the development of hallucinations, delusions, and/or

TABLE 3-1. **Functional complaints common to normal elderly persons**

Complaint	Comment
Sleep disturbance	Reduced total sleep time Increased sleep latency More frequent awakenings More time spent in bed Reduced "sleep efficiency"
Reduced appetite	Reduced energy expenditure Reduced activity Exacerbated by diminished taste and olfactory sensation, poor dentition, or unappealing diet
Reduced energy, fatigue	Exacerbated by chronic illness, especially obstructive lung disease and heart failure Also exacerbated by beta-blockers, clonidine, alphamethyldopa, anticonvulsants, and benzodiazepines
Impaired concentration and memory	Normal forgetfulness may be experienced as a symptom Exacerbated by sensory losses, especially diminished vision and hearing Exacerbated by central anticholinergic medications

bizarre behavior. The clinician's task is rendered easier still when typical depressive delusions (i.e., "mood-congruent delusions") are present, or when there is a past history of mood disorder. More challenging are those patients in whom the presenting complaint, often registered by family members, is of a persecutory delusion accompanied by prominent behavior disturbance. The following cases are illustrative.

A 76-year-old woman changed apartments several times because she believed her neighbors were aware of her responsibility for the President's "losing his veto power," which was going to lead to a "communist takeover." The delusion had emerged in the course of a series of unsatisfactory transactions with an air conditioner repairman who had told the patient that, lacking proper parts, he would attempt to "jury-rig" something for her. By the time she was hospitalized, her thinking was extremely disorganized and the term *jury-rigged* had acquired magical significance, with her failure to grasp its meaning directly responsible for the President's downfall. Several days of treatment with high-potency neuroleptics were required before the patient was able to give the history of change in mood, loss of appetite and weight, and anhedonia that accompanied and to some extent preceded the onset of her delusion. She responded very well to treatment for depression.

Another 72-year-old woman was a chronic problem for neighbors and police, convinced as she was that men were following her and wanted to "put her in a car with a large dog that would attack and kill her." Although some control of her fear and her bizarre behavior was achieved with neuroleptics, complete amelioration of her symptoms did not occur until antidepressant treatment was initiated, at which time her mood also greatly improved.

Accurate diagnosis is also impeded when patients cannot or will not report hallucinations or express the content of delusions, and the diagnosis must rest on bizarre behavior or severe thought disorder. Near-catatonic behavioral withdrawal is one such particularly common type of bizarre behavior and is often accompanied by refusal to eat, to maintain personal grooming, or to take medications. In the absence of a previous history of psychosis, late-life presentation of this syndrome should be regarded as psychotic depression until proven otherwise.

MASKED DEPRESSION

The literature has long reflected awareness by clinicians that depression in the elderly can be "masked" by physical complaints (7). In this presentation, subjective complaints of mood changes per se are replaced by multiple somatic complaints. In the course of medical diagnosis and treatment, these complaints are found to be either unaccompanied by anatomical or physiological abnormalities or out of proportion to the severity of these abnormalities. The prevalence of this syndrome in the elderly is not known;

early estimates that masked depression accounted for up to one-half of all cases of depression are certainly too high and in part reflect the inclusion of symptoms that would currently be regarded as neurovegetative features of major depression. Identification of this syndrome is particularly difficult when it occurs in patients with somatic complaints that are associated with clear physical causes. As Lipowski (8) has pointed out, DSM-III-R (9) criteria are usually adequate to diagnose patients presenting in this way, but the clinician must be particularly sensitive to objective indicators of depressed mood and must investigate carefully to discern associated neurovegetative features of major depression. A relatively sharp historical increase in the number and severity of physical complaints at or around the time of onset of neurovegetative signs or the occurrence of physical symptoms that are bizarre and illogical or that are temporally linked to social stressors typically associated with mood changes can alert the clinician to the possibility of an "underlying" major depression.

A 90-year-old woman complained of "her arms and legs twisting" along with a feeling of "buzzing" from the top of her head radiating into her chest, abdomen, arms, and hands. She insisted that the symptoms reflected a "heart attack" and made frequent unproductive visits to her local emergency room. Careful interviewing revealed that onset of these symptoms was associated with marital conflict, and exacerbations tended to occur when marital tensions escalated. Over the long run, she responded well to psychotherapy but refused antidepressants. She eventually gained a modest degree of insight into the functional nature of her complaints.

This variant of major depression differs from somatization disorder with depressed mood in the number of physical symptoms, which is typically as high as 20 or more in somatization disorder; in the history, which is typically much more chronic and unremitting in somatization disorder; and in the presence of neurovegetative features of depression, which are typically not present in somatization disorder. Elderly patients with masked depression may vary considerably in their hypochondriacal preoccupation with physical symptoms. At one extreme they may be simultaneously disabled by but relatively indifferent to their symptoms, whereas at the other extreme they may have a near-delusional conviction that symptoms reflect life-threatening illness and may make a life-style of doctor and diagnostic-procedure shopping. Unfortunately, available data do not justify precise criteria for establishing the diagnosis of masked depression. One reasonable diagnostic approach is to use DSM-III-R criteria for major depression, modifying criterion A as follows:

> At least five of the following symptoms have been present during the same 2-week period and represent a change from previous functioning; at least one of the symptoms is either *1)* depressed mood, *2)* loss of interest or pleasure, or *3)* persistent physical symptoms that cannot be explained by structural or functional pathology, or that have a distinctly bizarre or unusual quality that is not consistent with any known medical diagnosis.

PSEUDODEMENTIA

This presentation, more precisely known as "the dementia syndrome of depression," has been intensively studied, and a large literature is now available to guide the clinician. One study of hospitalized depressed elderly patients (10) found that 12 of 55 (22%) scored below 23 on the Mini-Mental State Exam (MMSE), indicating clinically significant cognitive impairment. Patients with this syndrome may appear severely demented, with poor grooming, slumped posture, and poor eye contact dramatizing their considerable cognitive deficits on mental status examination. However, when formally tested, they virtually never perform at a level consistent with severe organic dementia. So, for example, scores below 12–14 on the MMSE are rare, whereas scores in the single digits always point to organic dementia. Similarly, patients with uncomplicated dementia syndrome of depression do not display grossly disordered behavior, such as attempting to eat pencils, or placing underwear over outerwear, or climbing into other patients beds, or picking at their clothing. When severely disturbed behavior of this type is seen in a patient who otherwise meets criteria for a mood disorder, the presence of underlying organic brain disease or superimposed delirium must be ruled out.

Differentiating dementia syndrome of depression from early dementia can be quite difficult. Patients with this condition often score in the moderately impaired range on cognitive mental status examination (e.g., 15–22 on the MMSE) and may perform poorly on more detailed intellectual and memory testing. Minor functional deficits, such as forgetting staff names or repetitive asking of questions, may also be observed. Table 3-2 lists features that can help differentiate the dementia syndrome of depression from organic dementia in troublesome cases. Because these guidelines have not been validated by prospective investigation, they should be applied cautiously.

Often it may be necessary to observe response to treatment before forming a firm opinion about the presence of the dementia syndrome of depression. In our own work in this area, we found that cognitively impaired elderly depressed patients respond as well to antidepressant therapy as those without cognitive impairment. However, a lengthier and more aggressive course of treatment was required to achieve equivalent improvement (10).

ANOREXIA

A less common presentation of major depression in the elderly is profound anorexia, which may occur in the absence of any other neurovegetative features of depression, and in the presence of what otherwise appears to be normal mood and affect. This form of major depression seems to occur mainly in the "old old" and is often accompanied by multiple chronic, often "endstage," medical illnesses. The typical clinical picture is of a visibly aged, deteriorated, dysphoric patient who has "given up" and, by refusing to eat, appears to be committing passive suicide. Hospitalization of such patients may be complicated by family discord around the issue of the patient's "right to quit"; similar ambivalence is not uncommon among treatment staff, who may be prone to engage in prolonged discussion of the appropriateness of hospitalization, the quality of life required to warrant aggressive treatment, etc. To be sure, in some patients, particularly those from non-Western cultures, this clinical picture is interpreted by friends and family as an indication of the patient's wish to be dead, and the rendering of treatment aimed at restoring appetite is regarded as an insult to the elderly patient. These and similar

TABLE 3-2. **Differences between pseudodementia and dementia**

	Pseudodementia	Dementia
Clinical course and history	1. Onset fairly well demarcated	1. Onset indistinct
	2. History short	2. History quite long before consultation
	3. Rapidly progressive	3. Early deficits often go unnoticed
	4. History of previous psychiatric difficulty or recent life crisis	4. Previous psychiatric problem or emotional crisis uncommon
Clinical behavior	1. Detailed, elaborate complaints of cognitive dysfunction	1. Little complaint of cognitive loss
	2. Little effort expended on examination items	2. Struggle with cognitive tasks
	3. Affective change often present	3. Usually apathetic with shallow emotions
	4. Behavior does not reflect cognitive loss	4. Behavior compatible with cognitive loss
	5. Rarely has exacerbation at night	5. Nocturnal accentuation of dysfunction common
Examination findings	1. Frequently answers "I don't know" before even trying	1. Usually will try on items
	2. Inconsistent memory loss for both recent and remote items	2. Memory loss for recent events worse than remote

TABLE 3-2. **Differences between pseudodementia and dementia** (continued)

	Pseudodementia	Dementia
	3. May have particular memory gaps	3. No specific memory gaps
	4. In general, performance is inconsistent	4. Rather consistently impaired performance

Source. Adapted from Strub RL, Black FW: Neurobehavioral Disorders: A Clinical Approach. Philadelphia, PA, FA Davis, 1988, p 171. With permission. Copyright 1988 FA Davis Company.

considerations notwithstanding, a reasonable proportion of patients in this category respond to antidepressant treatment with restoration of normal appetite, weight gain, and the emergence of a new "will to live."

BEHAVIORAL REGRESSION

In some cases, an elderly patient gradually becomes less physically and socially active, neglects personal hygiene and necessary medical treatment, loses contact with friends and family, allows the home environment to become disordered and filthy, and may discontinue marketing and begin to live off canned or otherwise easily obtained food. On mental status examination, subjective change in mood and anhedonia may be denied, and objective signs of depression may be quite minimal. Dementia is commonly suspected in such individuals, and mental status examination may reveal some of the features described earlier under "Pseudodementia." As above, response to antidepressant medications may be dramatic.

PATHOGENESIS

As is the case with mood disorders in general, the etiology of major depression in the elderly is not known. Organic causes such as medications, stroke, and hypothyroidism are discussed below under "Organic Depression" and in Chapter 7 under "Psychiatric Symptoms Related to Medical Illness."

PSYCHODYNAMICS OF DEPRESSION IN THE ELDERLY

Psychodynamic theories of depression originated with Freud's elaborations on the theories of Karl Abraham regarding psychopathological developments in the process of mourning. In Freud's conception, the image or concept of the lost object (which may be an abstract object, such as professional status) is eventually introjected and becomes part of the self. Subsequent rage at the object, for leaving, and for past hurts and disappointments, thereby becomes directed at the self. The resultant loss of self-esteem, guilt, and need for punishment form the core of the symptom complex of "pathological grief." Other analytic conceptualizations of geriatric depression focus on helplessness experienced by the ego in light of failed attempts to live up to one's ideals, and the narcissistic injuries inevitably associated with the functional declines of age.

Although psychoanalytic theories of depression have not emphasized late life, the relatively high frequency of losses confronting many older individuals lends a measure of pertinence to each of these dynamic approaches to geriatric depression. The interested reader is directed to a useful review by Blau (11).

COGNITIVE AND BEHAVIORAL MODELS OF DEPRESSION

Seligman's concept of "learned helplessness" offers a theoretical connection between certain unavoidable losses of later life, such as declines in physical vigor, sexual function, and general health, and the sensation of passive helplessness often expressed by elderly depressed patients. Similarly, cognitive theorists point to the interaction between these losses and subsequent enaction of deeply ingrained, stable thought "schemata" as resulting in negative self-perceptions, which in turn lead to depressed mood. Depression may also be reinforced by life-styles that contain few opportunities to experience pleasurable life events (12).

NEUROBIOLOGICAL THEORIES

Neurobiological theories of late-life depression are similar in their focus on central neurotransmitter function to those proposed to explain depression in middle age, with emphasis on the role of age-related reductions in brain concentrations of norepinephrine, serotonin, dopamine, and acetylcholine and age-related increases in brain concentrations of monoamine oxidase (13,14). More recent research on endogenous rhythms has noted the similarity between certain abnormalities found in depression (e.g., advances in the phase of circadian cortisol secretion, increased body temperature, decreased nocturnal secretion of melatonin and thyroid-stimulating hormone, changes in sleep architecture) and those observed in normal aging (15).

An attempt to synthesize behavioral, cognitive, cultural, and biologic factors into a comprehensive model of geriatric depression was made by Chaisson-Stewart (16), based on the work of Adolf Meyer and Sir Aubrey Lewis. Briefly summarized, her view is that depression in the elderly represents the final result of an interaction between biological and/or psychosocial stressors, and "defenses," which include both learned psychological and genetically determined psychobiological mechanisms, which have been variably weakened by age and age-related infirmity.

DIAGNOSIS

DIAGNOSTIC CRITERIA

The diagnosis of major depression in the elderly begins with a detailed history of the present illness, focusing on relatively abrupt changes in one or more neurovegetative functions. For example, the patient may report that his or her usual pattern of unsatisfactory sleep became noticeably worse around the time that feelings of hopelessness and apathy were first experienced. Similarly, the gradual decline in activity and appetite that had been occurring for quite a while may also have abruptly accelerated around the same time. Again, informants such as a spouse or a child, a board-and-care home operator, or the family physician can be invaluable in establishing the timing of these changes. Diagnostic criteria for major depression (DSM-III-R) are displayed in Table 3-3.

LABORATORY EVALUATION

Laboratory evaluation of the elderly patient with major depres-

TABLE 3-3. **Diagnostic criteria for major depressive episode**

A. At least five of the following symptoms have been present nearly every day during the same 2-week period and represent a change from previous functioning; at least one of the symptoms is either (1) depressed mood, or (2) loss of interest or pleasure.

(1) Depressed mood
(2) Markedly diminished interest or pleasure in activities
(3) Significant weight loss or weight gain when not dieting or decrease or increase in appetite
(4) Insomnia or hypersomnia
(5) Psychomotor agitation or retardation
(6) Fatigue or loss of energy
(7) Feelings of worthlessness or excessive or inappropriate guilt
(8) Diminished ability to think or concentrate, or indecisiveness
(9) Recurrent thoughts of death, recurrent suicidal ideation, or a suicide attempt or a specific plan for committing suicide

Source. Adapted with permission from American Psychiatric Association: Diagnostic and Statistical Manual of Mental Disorders, 3rd Edition, Revised. Washington, DC, American Psychiatric Association, 1987, p 222. Copyright 1987 The American Psychiatric Association.

sion is aimed at ruling out endogenous organic causes, such as hypothyroidism and adrenal insufficiency, and establishing the pretreatment baseline status of physiological systems likely to be affected by psychoactive medications. A recommended battery of tests with their justification is given in Table 3-4.

Several more sophisticated laboratory procedures have been reported to be useful in establishing or ruling out a diagnosis of major depression. These include the dexamethasone suppression test (DST), the thyroid-releasing hormone (TRH) test, and the sleep electroencephalogram (SEEG). Details of the procedure of administration and relevant statistics for each of these tests can be found in the suggested readings at the end of this chapter and in Reference 17. Unfortunately, the rate of false positives and negatives for both the DST and the TRH test is so high in elderly patients, and the diagnostic confidence associated with these tests is, by virtue of depending on the underlying base rate (i.e., prevalence) of major depression, so unpredictable, that neither test is

TABLE 3-4. **Screening laboratory tests for evaluation of depression in the elderly**

Test	Potential diagnosis
Complete blood count with differential white count	Folate deficiency anemia, viral infection
Serum thyroid-stimulating hormone (TSH), thyroxine (T_4), serum cortisol (A.M. and P.M.)	Hypo-, hyperthyroidism; hypo-, hyperadrenocorticalism
Urinalysis, blood urea nitrogen	Uremia
SMA-18 (Sequential Medical Analysis—18)	Hypercalcemia, hypokalemia, hyperglycemia
Computed tomography or magnetic resonance imaging of head (as indicated by results of above tests, physical examination)	Brain tumor, stroke

recommended for routine clinical purposes. The SEEG, on the other hand, appears to be acceptably reliable, demonstrating increased percentage of rapid eye movement (REM) sleep, a longer first REM period, shorter REM latency (period of time of non-REM sleep before the first REM episode), and increased density of phasic eye movements in elderly depressed patients as compared with nondepressed, age-matched control subjects (18). However, the SEEG has yet to be shown to increase diagnostic accuracy beyond that of the clinical evaluation alone and is too expensive to be of widespread clinical utility.

RATING SCALES FOR DEPRESSION

Although depression rating scales were originally designed for research purposes, use of such scales in clinical practice can enhance uniformity and reliability of assessment. Symptom rating scales are not sufficient to establish a diagnosis of depression, but they can help to identify individuals whose depressive symptoms exceed the norm and can provide a means of tracking treatment-related change. We have found three depression scales to be clinically useful: the Beck Depression Inventory (BDI) (19), the Geriatric Depression Scale (GDS) (20), and the Hamilton Rating Scale for Depression (HAM-D) (21).

The BDI and the GDS are both self-rated instruments. The BDI is particularly useful for assessing psychological features of depression, including dysphoric mood, pessimism, self-criticism, and guilt. It is recommended for tracking symptom severity in older persons with relatively clear-cut depression that is not complicated by psychosis or prominent somatization. It may also help to distinguish normal bereavement from major depression, because bereaved individuals would not be expected to obtain high scores on items evaluating guilt, self-criticism, or risk of suicide. A cutoff score of 10 or higher has proved useful in screening applications with geriatric populations. The following is a sample item from this scale:

1. (0) I do not feel sad.
   (1) I feel sad.
   (2) I am sad all the time and I can't snap out of it.
   (3) I am so sad or unhappy I can't stand it.

The GDS was developed specifically for older adults, and a yes-no format is used to simplify the self-rating procedure for this population. Mood is extensively surveyed, and there are items assessing cognitive complaints and social behavior; by contrast, most somatic items have been eliminated from the GDS to prevent inflation of scores due to normal aging changes. The GDS has also been shown to be reliable and valid in clinical research with elderly medical and psychiatric patients. In the short-form version summarized in Table 3-5, a score of 5 or higher is recommended in screening for depression.

Self-rating scales may not be appropriate for some elderly patients, particularly those with visual deficits, limited education, poor English language proficiency, psychosis, or masked depression. An observer-rated instrument, such as the HAM-D, can be useful in these situations. Observer ratings may also be used in conjunction with patient ratings to obtain a more complete view

TABLE 3-5. Geriatric Depression Scale (short form)

Choose the best answer for how you felt over the past week

1. Are you basically satisfied with your life? Yes/No
2. Have you dropped many of your activities and interests? Yes/No
3. Do you feel that your life is empty? Yes/No
4. Do you often get bored? Yes/No
5. Are you in good spirits most of the time? Yes/No
6. Are you afraid that something bad is going to happen to you? Yes/No
7. Do you feel happy most of the time? Yes/No
8. Do you often feel helpless? Yes/No
9. Do you prefer to stay at home, rather than going out and doing new things? Yes/No
10. Do you feel you have more problems with memory than most? Yes/No
11. Do you think it is wonderful to be alive now? Yes/No
12. Do you feel pretty worthless the way you are now? Yes/No
13. Do you feel full of energy? Yes/No
14. Do you feel that your situation is hopeless? Yes/No
15. Do you think that most people are better off than you are? Yes/No

The following answers count 1 point; scores >5 indicate probable depression:

1. NO	6. YES	11. NO
2. YES	7. NO	12. YES
3. YES	8. YES	13. NO
4. YES	9. YES	14. YES
5. NO	10. YES	15. YES

Source. From Yesavage J, Brink T, Rose T, et al: Development and validation of a geriatric depression screening scale. J Psychiatr Res 17:37–49, 1983.

of symptom presentation or change. The HAM-D is weighted toward the types of symptoms that antidepressant medications would be expected to alter early in the course of treatment (e.g., sleep, weight change, psychomotor speed), although it also taps depressive mood, anxiety, and other psychological features. Several different cutoff scores have been used in the literature, but we have found scores of 16 or higher to be best for detecting significant depression when the 21-item scale is used. A structured interview guide has recently been published that may help to increase interrater reliability of the HAM-D (22). The following is a sample item from this scale:

Depressed Mood

(rate)
    0 = Absent
    1 = These feeling states indicated only on questioning
    2 = These feeling states spontaneously reported verbally
    3 = Communicates feeling states nonverbally—i.e., through facial expression, posture, voice and tendency to weep
    4 = Patient reports VIRTUALLY ONLY these feeling states in his spontaneous verbal and nonverbal communication.

Yesavage (23) and Gallagher (24) provide excellent reviews of these and other potentially useful scales. Clinicians are advised to become familiar with one or two scales at most and to use these consistently.

PSYCHOLOGICAL TESTS

Table 3-6 lists some of the psychological assessment procedures that may be useful with older patients whose depressive symptoms are complicated or unclear. Psychodiagnostic tests document current mood, thought patterns, and social tendencies and, in some circumstances, can suggest personality features that may affect the presentation of major depression. For example, a Minnesota Multiphasic Personality Inventory (MMPI) profile in which elevations on the hysteria or hypochondriasis scales are combined with depressive symptoms is frequently observed in individuals with masked depression.

For older patients who present with a combination of depressive and cognitive symptoms, a referral for neuropsychological testing is sometimes appropriate. Such testing provides a detailed survey of cognitive functions, which is compared with normative values for healthy older people and patient populations with depression or dementia (see Chapter 5). If an individual's scores closely approximate those of other depressed patients, neuropsychological findings might serve to strengthen a clinical impression of depressive pseudodementia.

DIFFERENTIAL DIAGNOSIS

Normal Bereavement

The findings of several studies generally agree that uncomplicated bereavement may include any or all of the features of major
depression except suicidality, psychosis, severe loss of self-esteem
and/or functionality, and psychomotor retardation. Appetite and
sleep disturbance, multiple somatic complaints, anhedonia, anxiety, mild feelings of self-deprecation, the passive wish to "join the
loved one," and sadness and other dysphoric moods are common,
but are generally less severe than in major depression.

Depressed patients are more prone to focus on themselves
and their role in the loss and consequently are more likely to feel
guilt and reduced self-esteem than normal mourners, who tend to
think more of the lost object (25). One series of studies found that
35% of a group of 109 bereaved widows aged an average of 61
years were depressed 1 month after the death of their spouse, but
that only 17% remained depressed after 13 months; moreover, the
best predictor was depression itself: 75% of those depressed at 13
months were depressed at 1 month (26,27).

In another series of studies, Parkes, Glick, and associates
(28–30) were able to discern rough "stages" of normal bereavement: an initial period of numbness, shock, disbelief, and empti-
ness, often accompanied by intense anxiety, sleep disturbance,
and somatic complaints, occurs for the first few weeks after the
death of the loved one. This is followed by a period of adjustment
lasting about 1 year, during which cognitive and affective "working through" occurs via a process of recollection, fantasy, and
rationalization. This phase is completed when acceptance occurs
and is followed by the third recovery phase in which "redefini-
tion" of self without the lost loved one occurs. Synthesizing the
above studies, it is clear that, although the time course of uncomplicated bereavement in the individual patient remains fairly
variable, the majority of bereaved elderly patients should be at or
clearly moving toward baseline status by the end of the 1st year.

Organic Mood Syndrome

Organic mood syndrome is defined in DSM-III-R as "prominent
and persistent depressed ... mood, resembling ... a Major

TABLE 3-6. **Psychological tests for geriatric depression**

Type of test	Name of test	Description	Indications/ contraindications	Outcome	Comment
Objective personality	Minnesota Multiphasic Personality Inventory (MMPI)	Self-rated questionnaire	Helps establish differential diagnosis, severity of depression, presence of suicidality. May detect masked depression/ uncooperative or confused patient.	Personality profile, estimate of response bias, diagnostic impression.	Short and oral forms available.
	Millon Clinical Multiaxial Inventory (MCMI)	Self-rated questionnaire	Same as for MMPI.	Same as for MMPI.	Anchored to DSM-III personality disorder categories: newer than MMPI and used mainly in younger adults to

Projective personality				
Rorschach inkblot test	Patient describes complex, unfamiliar patterns.	Same as for MMPI but also valuable to assess possible thought disorder. Useful for patients unaware of or unwilling to admit psychiatric problems.	Description of prominent concerns, thought patterns, and pathological tendencies.	Many older adults reluctant to respond, see test as too ambiguous. May give too few responses to score. Test particularly difficult to some and may be expensive.
Thematic apperception test (TAT)	Patient makes up stories for pictures of people in different situations.	Same as for MMPI and Rorschach, also reveals interpersonal concerns and habits.	Same as for Rorschach.	Geriatric version is available.

Depressive Episode, that is due to a specific organic factor" (9, p. 111) Diagnostic criteria require, in addition to mood disturbance as described above, "evidence from the history, physical examination, or laboratory tests of a specific organic factor (or factors) judged to be etiologically related to the disturbance" (p. 112). The diagnosis of organic mood syndrome is not made during the course of delirium. Although this definition and criteria set is significantly less detailed and more broad than those given for major depression, organic mood syndrome in the elderly can mimic in all respects the picture of functional major depression, including suicidality and psychosis. The most important diagnostic procedure is a careful drug-ingestion history, as drug-induced depression is probably the most common variety of organic mood syndrome. Whereas the requirement that mood disturbance be "due to" a specific organic factor would require knowledge beyond the present "state of the art" in psychiatry, a clear history of mood disorder occurring within days or weeks of commencing regular ingestion of any of the medications listed in Table 3-7 is adequate presumptive evidence to justify discontinuation, where medically feasible, of the suspected agent.

> A 75-year-old woman with no previous history of mood disorder complained of "waves of doom" coming over her and fearfully described "crazy" thoughts of suicide. She had lost almost 20 pounds in the preceding 4–6 weeks and came to psychiatric attention when her dermatologist found her "weeping in his waiting room." Careful questioning revealed that she had been started on the beta-blocker nadolol for a minor cardiac dysrhythmia about 3 weeks before the onset of symptoms. All symptoms disappeared with no specific treatment within 1 week of discontinuing the medication. Of note is the fact that, by virtue of its relatively low lipid solubility, nadolol has been claimed to be safer in this respect than the "first-generation" beta-blockers like propranolol.

Organic mood syndrome can also be caused by endogenous illnesses such as stroke or endocrinologic or electrolyte abnormalities; these syndromes are discussed in Chapter 7.

Dysthymic Disorder

Dysthymic disorder in adults as described in DSM-III-R is a chronic depression of mood (at least 2 years duration) that is

TABLE 3-7. **Medications that can cause depression**

- **Analgesics**
  Narcotics, including synthetics, e.g.,
    codeine
    meperidine (Demerol hydrochloride)
    morphine
    pentazocine (Talwin)
  Nonsteroidal anti-inflammatory agents, including,
    ibuprofen (Motrin)
    indomethacin (Indocin)
    naproxen (Naprosyn)

- **Antihypertensive agents**
  clonidine (Catapres)
  guanethidine (Ismelin)
  alpha-methyldopa (Aldomet)
  propranolol (Inderal)
  reserpine (various trade names)

- **Antipsychotic agents, including**
  chlorpromazine (Thorazine)
  fluphenazine (Prolixin)
  haloperidol (Haldol)
  molindone (Moban)
  thioridazine (Mellaril)
  thiothixene (Navane)

- **Anxiolytic agents, including**
  alcohol
  chlordiazepoxide (Librium)
  diazepam (Valium)
  lorazepam (Ativan)
  meprobamate (Miltown)
  oxazepam (Serax)

- **Cancer chemotherapeutic agents**
  L-asparaginase
  dactinomycin
  cis-platinum
  o,p-DDD
  dacarbazine
  nitrogen mustard
  procarbazine
  tamoxifen
  vincristine

TABLE 3-7. **Medications that can cause depression**
(continued)

- **Sedative-hypnotics, including**
  ethchlorvynol (Placidyl)
  flurazepam (Dalmane)
  glutethimide (Doriden)
  methyprylon (Noludar)
  pentobarbital sodium (Nembutal)
  phenobarbital (various trade names)
  secobarbital sodium (Seconal sodium)
  temazepam (Restoril)
  triazolam (Halcion)

- **Miscellaneous**
  cimetidine (Tagamet)
  dexamethasone (Decadron)
  oral contraceptives
  prednisone
  ranitidine hydrochloride (Zantac)
  steroids
  thiazide diuretics

variably accompanied by associated symptoms of appetite disturbance, sleep disturbance, low energy or fatigue, low self-esteem, poor concentration or difficulty making decisions, and feelings of hopelessness. It occurs in about 1.8% of elderly individuals during any given month. Dysthymic disorder is similar to but less severe and more chronic than major depression and typically makes its first appearance in adolescence or early adulthood. Dysthymia may be preceded by a (nonmood) Axis I or Axis III disorder ("secondary dysthymia") or may occur as an isolated syndrome ("primary dysthymia"). Diagnostic differentiation between major depression and dysthymia is complicated by the requirement that major depression cannot be diagnosed at any time during the 2-year period of chronic depression. This criterion may be very difficult to document, especially in the elderly patient subject to exacerbations of physical illness associated with transient fluctuations of mood and neurovegetative function indistinguishable from those of major depression.

Partial treatment of major depression with anxiolytics alone, or with inadequate doses of antidepressants, can produce a syndrome symptomatically indistinguishable from dysthymia. This condition is properly termed major depression in partial remission (9) and is readily identifiable if an accurate treatment history is obtained.

Characterologic Depression

Characterologic depression, although not corresponding to any official DSM-III-R diagnosis, is sometimes used to describe elderly patients whose lifelong characteristic mood, as perceived by themselves and/or others, is depressed. They may also suffer episodes meeting criteria for more specific mood disorder, such as dysthymia or major depression, but even between such episodes are pessimistic, anhedonic, critical, and "unhappy." The precise nosological status of this syndrome is unclear, but it is likely to be associated with personality pathology, and in many cases, a formal diagnosis of personality disorder is indicated. Narcissistic, borderline, avoidant, and dependent personality disorders are most likely to be complicated by this chronic depressive pattern. Unfortunately, little is known about the epidemiology, clinical course, or treatment of this condition.

■ BIPOLAR MOOD DISORDER

Recent data support conventional estimates that about 10% of patients with major mood disorder are ultimately diagnosed as bipolar, and there is little reason to doubt that this ratio applies equally to elderly patients. However, first onset of hypomania or mania after age 65 is regarded as quite rare, despite published reports suggesting that "masked hypomania" may present as catatonia, agitated depression, paranoid psychosis, severe behavioral regression, dementia, and even delirium, and that, consequently, misdiagnosis of hypomania and mania in elderly patients may be relatively common.

CLINICAL PRESENTATION

Besides those listed above, other reported age-related variations in the presentation of hypomania and mania in the elderly include: *1)* episodes are longer and cycles occur more rapidly, *2)* euphoria is less common than anger and irritability, *3)* paranoid delusional content is more common than grandiosity, and *4)* response to treatment is less reliable.

PATHOGENESIS

PSYCHODYNAMIC THEORIES

Relatively little has been written about the psychodynamics of hypomania and mania in elderly patients per se. Early psychodynamic considerations about mania weighed the relative importance of predisposing personality characteristics versus precipitating events, with investigators such as Kraeplin influenced by what seemed to be an inconsistent relationship between manic episodes and external life events. Although the question remains open, the psychodynamic literature from that point has generally agreed on the primary importance of constitutional factors in the development of the illness. Analytic theorists beginning with Abraham attempted to understand these constitutional factors in terms of predisposing personality characteristics and the interplay of "classical" psychodynamic mechanisms. In this regard, Abraham saw mania as a psychic regression to a state of intense ambivalence directed toward love objects, reflected in behavior by primitive impulsiveness. Later theorists conceptualized mania as a defense and tended to see the manic personality as immature, egocentric, chronically depressed, dependent on others for self-esteem, and dominated by feelings of interpersonal competitiveness and envy. Generally, psychodynamic theories of mania have come to be seen as more relevant to shifts of mood in normal individuals and have largely been supplanted by neurobiological theories in attempts to understand frank hypomania and mania.

NEUROBIOLOGICAL THEORIES

As is true for depression, neurobiological theories of mania largely focus on postulated abnormalities in the amount and distribution of the central neurotransmitters dopamine, norepinephrine, serotonin, and acetylcholine, and research in the elderly per se is scant. The age-related changes in these substances described above have not yet led to any widely promulgated hypothesis relating these changes to neurotransmitter-mediated mechanisms underlying mania, and the same is true of more recent work relating mania and hypomania to disturbances in circadian, seasonal, and circamenstrual rhythms.

DIAGNOSIS

DIAGNOSTIC CRITERIA

DSM-III-R diagnostic criteria for manic episode are listed in Table 3-8.

LABORATORY EVALUATION

Laboratory evaluation of the elderly patient with mania or hypomania is aimed at ruling out endogenous organic causes, such as hyperthyroidism, and establishing the pretreatment baseline sta-

---

TABLE 3-8. **Diagnostic criteria for manic episode**

Note: A "manic syndrome" includes criteria A, B, and C below. A "hypomanic syndrome" includes criteria A and B, but not C.

A. A distinct period of abnormally and persistently elevated, expansive, or irritable mood, and,

B. At least three of the following symptoms:

  (1) Inflated self-esteem or grandiosity
  (2) Decreased need for sleep
  (3) More talkative than usual or pressure to keep talking
  (4) Flight of ideas or subjective experience that thoughts are racing
  (5) Distractibility
  (6) Increase in goal-directed activity or psychomotor agitation
  (7) Excessive involvement in pleasurable activities that have a high potential for painful consequences

C. Marked impairment in occupational functioning or in usual social activities or relationships with others, or need for hospitalization to prevent harm to self or others.

Source. Adapted with permission from American Psychiatric Association: Diagnostic and Statistical Manual of Mental Disorders, 3rd Edition, Revised. Washington, DC, American Psychiatric Association, 1987, p 217. Copyright 1987 The American Psychiatric Association.

tus of physiological systems likely to be affected by antimanic medications. A recommended battery of tests with their justification is given in Table 3-9.

DIFFERENTIAL DIAGNOSIS

Organic Mania

Mania or hypomania secondary to organic causes may be clinically indistinguishable from the functional variety. Endogenous illnesses that have been associated with the manic syndrome include hyperadrenocorticalism, hyperthyroidism, multiple sclerosis, brain tumor, and epilepsy. Exogenous causes include psychostimulants (amphetamines, methylphenidate, cocaine), tricyclic antidepressants, monoamine oxidase inhibitors, *L*-dopa, phencyclidine, alprazolam, and corticosteroids. In this regard, hypomania or mania that begins during chronic treatment with one or more of the above medications, but fails to resolve after discontinuation of the suspect medication(s), should be regarded as organically triggered rather than organically caused and should not be diagnosed as organic mania.

TABLE 3-9. **Laboratory evaluation of hypomania-mania in the elderly**

Test	Potential diagnosis
Blood studies	
Thyroid-stimulating hormone (TSH), thyroxine (T_4)	Hyperthyroidism
Cortisol (A.M. and P.M.)	Hyperadrenocorticalism
Sedimentation rate	Collagen-vascular disease, especially lupus
Lumbar puncture	Viral encephalitis
Computed tomography or magnetic resonance imaging of head	Brain tumor, stroke, multiple sclerosis

Mixed Mood Disorder

Elderly patients with major mood disorder commonly present with a syndrome of mixed manic and depressive features. A typical picture might include severe psychomotor agitation accompanied by intrusive and demanding behavior, irritability, flight of ideas and circumstantiality, anorexia, and insomnia. The question of whether agitated depression or mixed manic-depressive syndrome is the correct diagnosis can usually be resolved by applying DSM-III-R guidelines as listed above for bipolar disorder, mixed.

■ REFERENCES

1. Regier DA, Boyd JH, Burke JD, et al: One-month prevalence of mental disorders in the United States. Arch Gen Psychiatry 45:977–986, 1988

2. Blazer D, Williams C: Epidemiology of dysphoria and depression in an elderly population. Am J Psychiatry 137:439–444, 1980

3. Spar J, Ford CV, Liston EH: Hospital treatment of elderly neuropsychiatric patients, II: statistical profile of the first 122 patients in a new teaching ward. J Am Geriatr Soc 28:539–543, 1980

4. Gurland GJ, Cross PS: Epidemiology of psychopathology in old age. Psychiatr Clin North Am 5:11–26, 1982

5. Okimoto JT, Barnes RT, Veith RC, et al: Screening for depression in geriatric medical patients. Am J Psychiatry 139:799–802, 1982

6. Meyers BS, Greenberg R, Mei-Tal V: Delusional depression in the elderly, in Treatment of Affective Disorders in the Elderly. Edited by Shamoian CA. Washington, DC, American Psychiatric Press, 1985, pp 19–28

7. Kielholz P (ed): Masked Depression. Berne, H Huber, 1973

8. Lipowski ZJ: Somatization: the concept and its clinical application. Am J Psychiatry 145:1358–1368, 1988

9. American Psychiatric Association: Diagnostic and Statistical Manual of Mental Disorders, 3rd Edition, Revised. Washington, DC, American Psychiatric Association, 1987

10. LaRue A, Spar J, Dessonville Hill C: Cognitive impairment in late-life depression: clinical correlates and treatment implications. J Affect Disord 11:179–184, 1986

11. Blau D: Depression and the elderly: a psychoanalytic perspective, in Depression and Aging. Edited by Breslau LD, Haug MR. New York, Springer, 1983, pp 75–93

12. Gatz M, Popkin SJ, Pino CD, et al: Psychological interventions with older adults, in Handbook of the Psychology of Aging, 2nd Edition. Edited by Birren JE, Schaie KW. New York, Von Nostrand Reinhold, 1985, pp 669–685

13. Lipton MA: Age differentiation in depression: biochemical aspects. J Gerontol 31:293–298, 1976

14. Epstein LJ: Depression in the elderly. J Gerontol 31:278–282, 1976

15. Sack DA, Rosenthal NE, Parry BL, et al: Biological rhythms in psychiatry, in Psychopharmacology: The Third Generation of Progress. Edited by Meltzer HY. New York, Raven, 1987

16. Chaisson-Stewart GM: An integrated theory of depression, in Depression in the Elderly. Edited by Chaisson-Stewart GM. New York, John Wiley, 1985, pp 56–104

17. APA Task Force on Laboratory Tests in Psychiatry: The dexamethasone suppression test: an overview of its current status in psychiatry. Am J Psych 144:1253–1262, 1987

18. Reynolds CF, Kupfer DJ, Houck PR, et al: Reliable discrimination of elderly depressed and demented patients by electroencephalographic sleep data. Arch Gen Psychiatry 45:258–264, 1988

19. Beck AT: Depression Inventory. Philadelphia, PA, Philadelphia Center for Cognitive Therapy, 1978

20. Yesavage J, Brink T, Rose T, et al: Development and validation of a geriatric depression screening scale. J Psychiatr Res 17:37–49, 1983

21. Hamilton M: Rating depressive patients. J Clin Psychiatry 41:21–24, 1960

22. Williams JBW: A structured interview guide for the Hamilton Depression Rating Scale. Arch Gen Psychiatry 45:742–747, 1988

23. Yesavage JA: The use of self-rating depression scales in the elderly, in Handbook for Clinical Memory Assessment of Older Adults. Edited by Poon L. Washington, DC, American Psychological Association, 1986, pp 213–217

24. Gallagher D: Assessment of depression by interview methods and psychiatric rating scales, in Handbook for Clinical Memory Assessment of Older Adults. Edited by Poon L. Washington, DC, American Psychological Association, 1986, pp 202–213

25. Gallagher D, Breckenridge JN, Thompson LW, et al: Similarities and differences between normal grief and depression in older adults. Essence 5:127–140, 1982

26. Clayton PJ, Halikas JA, Maurice W: The depression of widowhood. Br J Psychiatry 120:71–78, 1972

27. Bornstein PE, Clayton PJ, Halikas JA, et al: The depression of widowhood after thirteen months. Br J Psychiatry 122:561–566, 1973

28. Parkes CM: Bereavement and mental illness, Part 2: classification of

bereavement reactions. Br J Med Psychol 38:13–26, 1965

29. Parkes CM: Bereavement: Studies of Grief in Adult Life. New York, International Universities Press, 1972

30. Glick IO, Weiss S, Parkes CM: The First Year of Bereavement. New York, John Wiley, 1974

■ ADDITIONAL READINGS

Beck JC (ed): Year Book of Geriatrics and Gerontology. Chicago, IL, Year Book, 1989

Storandt M: Counseling and Therapy With Older Adults. Boston, MA, Little, Brown, 1983

MOOD DISORDERS— TREATMENT

4

This chapter generally applies to treatment of major depression and its variants. Few guidelines are available in the geriatric literature to assist the clinician in the selection of treatment, although guidelines developed in the general psychiatric literature appear generally to hold for elderly patients as well. This literature suggests that psychosocial and somatic approaches are usually additive in effect and should be offered together wherever possible, as limited by social, financial, and clinical circumstances.

■ PSYCHOSOCIAL THERAPY

Individual, group, and family therapy, with or without concomitant administration of psychoactive medications, can be appropriate and effective interventions for the elderly patient with major depression.

INDIVIDUAL THERAPY

Individual psychotherapy is similar to that used for the middle-aged patient, with the following modifications. The therapist may need to be more active, to speak louder and more slowly, and to sit closer than would be appropriate with a younger patient. Sessions typically are shorter, and patients often require reminder calls; telephone contact per se is often a large part of the ongoing therapeutic relationship. Amplifying devices are often needed, and explanations may need to be more concrete and simple. Where possible, treatment goals and processes should be specified, and questions and concerns directly addressed (1).

Although cognitive, behavior, and psychodynamic therapies have all been demonstrated to be effective in the elderly depressive patient, the presence of neurovegetative signs, personality disorder, or low patient expectation of positive outcome all predict relatively poor outcome of these therapies when they are administered without concomitant somatic therapy (2). For obvious reasons, significant cognitive impairment and psychosis are relative contraindications for psychotherapy, although supportive individual therapy with such patients in the hospital may be useful per se and may maximize patient cooperation with somatic therapies.

The use of the psychotherapeutic relationship to facilitate ongoing evaluation of response to pharmacotherapy is an important function for individual therapy that has received little formal study. Because initiation and regulation of pharmacotherapy for major depression may take several months, the opportunity to accomplish significant psychotherapeutic work is presented even with patients who might otherwise be resistant to psychotherapy. In this regard, depressed patients with neurovegetative signs or psychosis, for whom the above-cited research suggests that psychotherapy alone may be ineffective, can benefit from therapy administered while adjusting dosages of antidepressant and antipsychotic medications.

GROUP THERAPY

As with individual therapy, several approaches have been demonstrated to be effective in depressed elderly patients (3). In general, standard methods, modified as above, are appropriate. Patient selection is particularly important with respect to organic mental impairment, sensory deficits, and physical illness, any of which may limit a patient's capacity to tolerate and benefit from group therapy and may negatively influence group process. Patients with moderate to severe deafness, cognitive impairment, psychosis, involuntary movements, pain, or dyspnea are relatively poor candidates for group therapy.

FAMILY THERAPY

Major depression commonly presents a crisis for families, particularly if a significant delay in diagnosis and administration of treatment occurs and significant deterioration of function is allowed to occur. By the time adequate medical attention is obtained, major disruption in the lives of two or three generations of the family has often taken place. Because family members are often required to provide details of medical and psychiatric history and are frequently involved in patient management (assisting with transportation, encouraging compliance with treatment, etc.), the family-therapy format is the preferred approach in many if not most cases. The family setting allows:

- Gathering of information about the patient from multiple perspectives at once.
- Efficient dissemination of information about the patient and his or her treatment plan.
- Assessment of family dynamics that may color such perspectives.
- The opportunity to address those family conflicts that have been precipitated by and may impede evaluation and treatment of the present crisis. Because of these advantages, family members should participate in treatment of the depressed older patient whenever possible.

■ SOMATIC THERAPY

This section will review the somatic treatment of nonpsychotic depression and its variants. Because the presence of psychosis (hallucinations, delusions, severe thought disorder, or behavioral regression) appears to significantly reduce the effectiveness of antidepressant therapy, even when concomitant antipsychotic medications are prescribed, this variant is discussed under a separate heading.

PSYCHOPHARMACOLOGY

The first line of psychopharmacologic treatment of nonpsychotic major depression in the elderly remains the cyclic antidepressants, all of which act, at least indirectly, by blocking central presynaptic reuptake of norepinephrine, serotonin, or both. Although the controlled-research literature is relatively sparse, these medications are roughly twice as effective as placebo in carefully selected elderly depressed patients (4). As there is little evidence of superior efficacy of one agent over another, the choice of first treatment is usually based on side-effect profiles, which are related to each agent's affinity for central muscarinic receptors (anticholinergic effects), histaminic (H1) receptors (drowsiness and appetite stimulation), and noradrenergic receptors (orthostatic hypotension) (Table 4-1). For this reason, the tertiary tricyclics (e.g., amitriptyline, imipramine, doxepin, trimipramine) are generally avoided, because they are significantly more sedating, anticholinergic, and prone to cause orthostatic hypotension than their demethylated counterparts, the secondary tricyclics (e.g., desipramine, nortriptyline, protriptyline), or certain of the nontricyclics (e.g., trazodone, fluoxetine hydrochloride). Tertiary tricyclics also are probably more likely to delay cardiac conduction (see below) than the secondary or nontricyclic agents.

Because of its relatively strong association with seizures, the tetracyclic maprotiline is not recommended as a first-line treatment, and because of its mixed neuroleptic-antidepressant properties and attendant risks of extrapyramidal symptoms and tardive dyskinesia, the dibenzoxazepine amoxapine is similarly not recommended as a first-line treatment. The above reasoning leaves desipramine, nortriptyline, protriptyline, trazodone, and fluoxetine as the preferred first-line cyclic antidepressants.

TABLE 4-1. **Cyclic antidepressant receptor affinities**

Agent	Daily dosage (mg)	H1 affinity[a]	α-1 affinity[b]	Muscarinic affinity[c]
Amitriptyline	75–150	91	3.7	5.5
Trimipramine	75–150	370	4.2	1.7
Doxepin	75–200	420	1.1	1.1
Imipramine	75–150	9	1.1	1.1
Nortriptyline	25–100	10	1.7	0.67
Protriptyline	15–40	4	0.77	4.0
Desipramine	75–200	0.91	0.77	0.50
Maprotiline	75–150	50	1.1	0.18
Amoxapine	75–300	4	2.0	0.10
Trazodone	150–300	0.29	2.8	0.00031

Note. All affinity units are $10^{-7} \times 1/K_d$, where K_d is the equilibrium dissociation constant in molarity.
[a]Approximately correlates with potential for appetite stimulation and sedation. [b]Approximately correlates with potential for orthostatic hypotension. [c]Approximately correlates with potential for anticholinergic symptoms.
Source. Adapted from Wise WG, Rundell JR: A Concise Guide to Consultation Psychiatry. Washington, DC, American Psychiatric Press, 1988, p 47. With permission from publisher. Copyright 1988 American Psychiatric Press.

CYCLIC ANTIDEPRESSANTS

Desipramine

Advantages. Desipramine has a low side-effect profile, is activating, and is generally well tolerated. In nonelderly adults, desipramine appears to have a roughly linear serum level–response relationship (i.e., no "therapeutic window"), with the likelihood of response increasing as serum levels rise above 115 ng/ml (5). Although one naturalistic pilot study in 22 elderly depressed patients of average age 71.3 years found the effective serum level to be about one-half that amount (6), our clinical experience is more consistent with the higher figure. Another potential advantage of desipramine is that response may be predicted by a methylphenidate challenge (see below).

Disadvantages. Of the secondary tricyclics, desipramine is not as well studied as nortriptyline, particularly in patients with cardiac conduction disturbance and congestive heart failure, and is therefore possibly not as safe; one study reported modest prolongation of cardiac conduction in 10 elderly depressed patients who had therapeutic desipramine levels (i.e., between 125 and 300 ng/ml) (7). As a purely noradrenergic agent, it may be less effective in patients whose depression responds better to a mixed noradrenergic-serotonergic agent, such as nortriptyline.

Nortriptyline

Advantages. Nortriptyline is of demonstrated safety in patients with congestive heart failure (i.e., produces somewhat less orthostatic hypotension) and is probably less likely than desipramine to prolong cardiac conduction in therapeutic dosage ranges. One study suggests that a single 25-mg test dose can predict the final dosage necessary to attain therapeutic serum levels (8).

Disadvantages. Nortriptyline probably has a "therapeutic window" (estimated to fall between 50 and 150 ng/ml) such that serum levels above or below that range are relatively ineffective. Accordingly, relatively slow dosage increases and or serum level monitoring are required.

Protriptyline

Advantages. The most activating of the tricyclic agents, protriptyline may be particularly useful in patients with severe psychomotor retardation and/or Parkinson's disease.

Disadvantages. Protriptyline is not well studied, and therefore effects in patients with congestive heart failure or cardiac conduction disturbance have not been well characterized. Also, the serum level–response relationship has not been studied.

Trazodone

Advantages. Trazodone has no anticholinergic effects, is probably less likely to prolong cardiac conduction, and is therefore a good treatment for patients with bundle branch block (9).

Disadvantages. Trazodone is extremely sedating, may cause mild gastrointestinal upset, and produces orthostatic hypotension. Unpublished data support the clinical observation that, although the absolute rate of remission produced by trazodone is similar, response is more yes/no than with tricyclic antidepressants, which tend to produce some improvement in patients who do not sustain complete remission.

Fluoxetine

Advantages. Fluoxetine has mild psychostimulant-like effects and is only weakly anticholinergic. Cardiac effects are unclear but probably minimal. The recommended initial and final dosage of 20 mg (except in the rare nonresponder who may require up to 60 mg per day) eliminates the need to gradually increase the dose and simplifies the "induction phase" of therapy.

Disadvantages. Fluoxetine may interfere with sleep and appetite. Early clinical experience with lithium augmentation (elderly patients on 20 mg per day of fluoxetine) has resulted in three cases of severe, gross intention/action tremor that developed within several days of initiating lithium therapy and disappeared within several days of its discontinuation. Although the tremor was reversible, it was severe enough to make eating or drinking impossible without assistance. To date, this effect has not been described in the literature and may not be typical.

General Principles of Treatment With Cyclic Antidepressants

Pretreatment evaluation. Before initiating cyclic antidepressant therapy in an older patient, the following procedures are recommended:

- *Physical and neurological examination.* Specifically oriented toward detection of signs of narrow-angle glaucoma, prostatism, and xerostomia, all of which may be aggravated by anticholinergic effects of tricyclics, and congestive heart failure, which may predispose to the development of significant orthostatic hypotension.
- *Measurement of orthostatic change in blood pressure.* Pretreatment orthostatic hypotension may predispose to worsening with treatment, possibly leading to dizziness and falls. Some evidence has been gathered that patients who demonstrate relatively greater magnitude of orthostatic fall in systolic blood pressure may respond better to treatment (see below).
- *Electrocardiogram* (12 lead). Obtained primarily to determine the presence of cardiac conduction disturbance. Although recent research indicates that bundle branch block presents the greatest risk for development of complete heart block, caution is also recommended in patients who demonstrate first-degree block (i.e., prolonged P-R interval) as well as prolonged QRS interval. Other potentially important findings include sick sinus syndrome, which precludes administration of lithium salts, and supraventricular arrythmia, which could be aggravated by anticholinergic effects of tricyclics.
- *Liver function tests* (e.g., bilirubin, serum glutamic-oxaloacetic transaminase [SGOT], serum glutamic pyruvic transaminase [SGPT], alkaline phosphatase). Significant hepatic disease is a relative contraindication for use of tricyclics and may lead to very high serum levels and possible toxicity.

Predictors of response. A few published studies have examined procedures for predicting which elderly depressed patients will respond to treatment with cyclic antidepressants. Research in middle-aged adults suggesting that a positive dexamethasone suppression test (DST) is a predictor of good response to somatic therapy has generally not been replicated in elderly populations; indeed, one inpatient study of depressed elderly patients concluded that a positive DST was a marker of greater severity and poorer response to somatic therapy (10). Several studies of elderly depressive patients have suggested that pretreatment orthostatic decrease in systolic blood pressure is associated with a better outcome of treatment: patients with a decrease greater than 10–12 mmHg had better response to treatment with tricyclic antidepressants than those with a decrease of less than 10 mmHg (11,12). Because orthostatic blood pressure as measured by a simple blood pressure cuff technique is affected by many factors and tends to be an inherently unstable measure, it is difficult to explain these findings at present. Another study found that a 20-mg oral dose of methylphenidate was useful in predicting outcome of treatment with desipramine in elderly depressed inpatients. Those whose mood failed to improve within 1–2 hours of ingestion of methylphenidate tended to respond less well to desipramine than those who did improve after methylphenidate (13). However, this was an uncontrolled study that has not yet been replicated.

Initiation of therapy. In general, starting dosages should be small: 25–50 mg of desipramine or nortriptyline, 50–75 mg of trazodone, 20 mg of fluoxetine. Compliance is usually enhanced by minimizing the number of doses administered during any 24-hour period. In this regard, all of the agents in this category have roughly a 24-hour or greater half-life and can be given in a single bedtime dosage except fluoxetine, which is administered in the morning, and trazodone, which has a shorter half-life but can be successfully administered in a single bedtime dosage anyway. For patients who get up at night (e.g., to urinate), this may present problems, because peak serum levels will occur when the patient is least careful to arise slowly, ambulate carefully, etc. Also, some patients experience psychomotor activation with nortriptyline or desipramine and suffer impaired sleep after bedtime doses.

Determination of final dose. The most common cause of treatment failure with antidepressants is inadequate dosage, which typically causes side effects while effecting only partial or no symptom remission, thereby leaving patients worse off than without treatment. Therefore, it is important to gradually increase dosages until each patient's ceiling, determined by the development of side effects, has been reached, or remission is adequate. With nortriptyline only, this strategy risks passing through the "therapeutic window," so plasma level determination may be necessary in the nonresponder. With other agents, plasma levels offer little clinically relevant information in most cases and are not obtained. However, in the unusual patient in whom very low dosages produce unexpectedly intense side effects, or very high dosages fail to produce side effects or mood elevation, determination of plasma level may be useful. Therapeutic levels as determined by study of geriatric subjects per se are unclear, but in general, higher levels are associated with better outcome.

Management of side effects. The most dangerous side effect of tricyclic antidepressant therapy in the elderly is orthostatic hypotension. This symptom tends to occur early in treatment and appears to be a "threshold" phenomenon that appears at a certain dosage but does not necessarily worsen if the dosage is increased. Because it is worsened by dehydration and by pooling of blood in the lower extremities, it can be ameliorated by increasing salt in the patient's diet, or by administration of small doses of salt-retaining steroids (e.g., .025–.05 mg of fluorohydrocortisone). Support hose can be helpful, as can careful, repeated patient instruction in arising slowly and holding on to something stable for support. Anticholinergic effects of tricyclics include dry mouth, constipation, blurry vision, urinary hesitancy, and central anticholinergic delirium. Dry mouth is relieved by sucking on hard, preferably sugarless candies, or by chewing gum. A 1% solution of pilocarpine used as a mouthwash every 3 or 4 hours has also been reported to be helpful (14). Constipation can be managed with stool softeners, bulk laxatives, and adequate fluid intake. Blurry vision may respond to 1% pilocarpine eye drops, one drop every 4–6 hours as needed. In milder cases, artificial tears usually suffice. Urinary hesitancy is often responsive to oral bethanechol, 10–30 mg 3 times a day. Patients, particularly men, are instructed to be aware of the possibility of complete urinary obstruction and to have appropriate plans should complete obstruction occur (e.g., to report to the nearest emergency room).

Delirium can be life threatening and is usually responsive to discontinuation of the offending agent and supportive treatment. In the extreme case, 1–2 mg of physostigmine administered by slow intravenous push is effective. Of the cyclic antidepressants, trazodone is the only agent essentially free of anticholinergic side effects and may be the treatment of first choice for patients with unusual sensitivity to the above side effects.

MONOAMINE OXIDASE INHIBITORS

Monoamine oxidase inhibitors (MAOIs), which inhibit synaptic degradation of the monoamine neurotransmitters (including norepinephrine and serotonin), have not been as well studied in elderly patients as the cyclic antidepressants, but enjoy widespread clinical use and appear to be as effective as the cyclic antidepressants (15). Controlled studies demonstrating particular effectiveness of MAOIs in so-called atypical depression, characterized by high levels of anxiety and hypochondriasis, hyperphagia, and hypersomnolence have not been replicated in elderly subjects per se, and until such studies are published, the specificity of MAOIs in the elderly remains undefined.

In the United States, phenelzine, tranylcypromine, and isocarboxazid are available for treatment of depression (pargyline, a monoamine oxidase–inhibiting antihypertensive agent, will not be discussed here). Effective dosages are 15 mg twice per day, gradually increased to a maximum of 60–75 mg per day for phenelzine, 10 mg twice per day increasing to a maximum of 50 mg per day for tranylcypromine, and 10 mg twice per day increasing to a maximum of 30 mg per day for isocarboxazid. All three agents are relatively free of sedative and anticholinergic effects and do not appear to affect cardiac conduction. All three cause orthostatic hypotension, however, and in the presence of sympathomimetic drugs, dietary monoamine precursors such as tryptophan, or naturally occurring pressor substances such as tyramine can cause severe hypertensive reactions that can be life threatening. Orthostatic hypotension from MAOIs is somewhat different from that produced by cyclic antidepressants in that it tends to be dose related, occurs later in therapy, and may gradually subside at a fixed dosage.

Phenelzine

Advantages. Phenelzine is nonstimulating and may be mildly sedating.

Disadvantages. Phenelzine causes irreversible degradation of monoamine oxidase and therefore may continue to exert effects for 2 weeks or longer after discontinuation of administration, as total body monoamine oxidase is gradually replaced.

Tranylcypromine

Advantages. Tranylcypromine is mildly stimulating and may be preferable for patients with psychomotor retardation. It is reversibly bound to monoamine oxidase and therefore requires only a 1-week washout period before sympathomimetic agents or diet ad libitum can be administered safely.

Disadvantages. Because of its psychostimulant effects, tranylcypromine may have greater abuse potential.

Isocarboxazid
See remarks as for phenelzine above.

General Principles of Treatment With MAOIs

Pretreatment evaluation. Physical and laboratory evaluation should be conducted as described above for cyclic antidepressants. Determination of pretreatment orthostatic change in blood pressure should be performed before initiating treatment with MAOIs. Based on the above procedures and the medical history, the patient's likelihood of requiring sympathomimetic agents must also be assessed. Elderly patients with chronic asthma or bronchitis who must be treated with bronchodilators or patients with Parkinson's disease who may require treatment with L-dopa are not candidates for MAOI therapy.

Based on the above procedures, the medical and social history, and the current living situation, the patient's reliability vis-à-vis dietary and medication restrictions must be carefully assessed. Specifically, patients who are mildly demented or worse, and who are monitoring their own diet and medications, are poor candidates for MAOI therapy.

Initiation of therapy. Typical starting dosages are 15 mg twice a day for phenelzine and 10 mg twice a day for isocarboxazid and tranylcypromine.

Determination of final dosage. As per the cyclic antidepressants, optimal response depends on adequate dosage. Although it has been demonstrated in nongeriatric subjects that platelet monoamine oxidase inhibition must reach 80% or more to maximize response, in clinical practice this laboratory test is rarely available, and maximum tolerable dosage or clear clinical response remains the end point of dosage titration. Practically speaking, most elderly patients experience dosage-limiting orthostatic hypotension at or before 60 mg per day of phenelzine, 40 mg per day of tranylcypromine, or 30 mg per day of isocarboxazid.

Management of side effects. Orthostatic hypotension may be managed via the approaches described above for cyclic antidepressants. Hypertensive crisis is usually signaled by headache, flushing, diaphoresis, and palpitations and may progress to frank hypertensive encephalopathy and neurologic dysfunction. α-Adrenergic blocking agents such as phentolamine (2–5 mg iv) or chlorpromazine (50–100 mg im) followed by smaller doses titrated against blood pressure may be lifesaving. The common practice of giving patients a 50- or 100-mg tablet of chlorpromazine to carry with them for ingestion in an emergency has been criticized on the grounds that after ingestion many older patients may be so incapacitated as to be unable to reach the nearest emergency room or may experience life-threatening loss of alertness while driving for help.

Special considerations. A particular hazard is the use of sympathomimetic drug–containing cold tablets and nasal sprays (e.g., ephedrine, pseudoephedrine, phenylephrine [Neo-Synephrine], phenylpropanolamine), which may not be regarded as "real medicine" by older patients. These must be cautioned against most strenuously. Meperidine, for reasons that are not yet clear, interacts with MAOIs to produce an extremely serious syndrome of hyperpyrexia, muscular rigidity, and coma that has been fatal in several reported instances. Other synthetic narcotics such as dextromethorphan have also been implicated in causing this syndrome, which apparently does not occur with natural narcotics such as morphine or codeine. For added safety, patients may wear "medical alert" bracelets indicating that they are on MAOIs and specifying that they should not receive meperidine. Similarly, dental procedures should be performed with local anesthetics that do not contain epinephrine.

LITHIUM SALTS

Although there is no controlled-research literature on the use of lithium as a treatment for geriatric depression per se (i.e., in patients with major depression with or without bipolar mood disorder), studies in middle-aged patients suggest that lithium alone is significantly superior to placebo for this indication. Given the exquisite sensitivity of many older patients to the side effects of cyclic antidepressants and MAOIs, this area of therapeutics deserves systematic investigation by clinicians and researchers.

General Principles of Treatment With Lithium Salts

Pretreatment evaluation. Before initiating lithium therapy in the older patient, the following procedures are recommended:

- *Physical and neurological examination.* Specifically oriented toward detection of thyroid enlargement, evidence of renal dysfunction, and tremor, all of which may be exacerbated by lithium therapy. Evidence of congestive heart failure, which may require initiation of diuretic therapy, is particularly important because diuretics can significantly increase lithium blood levels.
- *Electrocardiogram.* Evidence of sinus node dysfunction (sick sinus syndrome) is a strong relative contraindication for lithium therapy because significant bradycardia or dysrhythmia may be precipitated. Benign nonspecific T wave abnormalities that reverse with cessation of treatment are common in patients taking lithium and do not require discontinuation of treatment.
- *Laboratory evaluation.* Laboratory evaluation is oriented toward detection of renal dysfunction, i.e., serum creatinine, blood urea nitrogen, electrolytes, and establishment of pretreatment thyroid function (triiodothyronine [T_3], thyroxine [T_4]). Because lithium therapy can effect thyroid function, periodic (e.g., every 6 months) physical examination of the thyroid and reevaluation of serum T_3 and T_4 is recommended.

Initiation of therapy and determination of final dosage. Elderly patients generally require smaller dosages of lithium to reach therapeutic serum levels and may require lower serum levels for therapeutic effect. Therefore, initial doses are small (e.g., 150 mg twice a day) and are titrated upward to achieve serum levels in the 0.6–1.0 meq/ml range for treatment of hypomania or mania, or 0.3–0.7 meq/ml for prophylaxis. Serum for determination of lithium level is drawn after 4–5 days at a steady daily dosage, and a roughly linear dosage–serum level relationship is assumed within therapeutic dosage ranges.

Because clinical response and side effects can occur at any serum level, these ranges are only valuable as rough clinical guidelines.

Management of side effects. Acute side effects include nausea, diarrhea, mild polydipsia and polyuria, and generalized fine tremor. Nausea can be minimized by administering doses after meals, and by preceding doses with prophylactic antacids. Diarrhea is usually mild and intermittent and rarely may require concomitant antidiarrheal therapy. Tremor is not usually of clinical significance and rarely requires dosage manipulation. Side effects of chronic therapy may include hypothyroidism and goiter, and the question of renal tubular damage remains controversial.

PSYCHOSTIMULANTS

Although there are few controlled studies, several recent clinical reports support the use of psychostimulants in elderly depressed patients, particularly those in whom medical illness precludes the use of cyclic or MAOI antidepressants. Amphetamines and methylphenidate have both been recommended, although methylphenidate is generally preferred because of its relatively lower cardiovascular side-effect profile. Dosages range from 5 to 20 mg administered orally twice a day, generally immediately before breakfast and lunch so as not to interfere with appetite or sleep. Cardiovascular side effects are typically limited to very minor increases in blood pressure and heart rate. The most common side effect is mild "jitteriness," which may be managed with small doses of benzodiazepine anxiolytics, but severe dysphoria and agitation, appetite disturbance, and insomnia requiring discontinuation of treatment may occur in the rare patient.

There seem to be several patterns of response: acute mood elevation after the first few doses only, with rapid loss of effect thereafter; subacute mood elevation that deteriorates after a few weeks despite dosage increase; and sustained (i.e., for months or years) mood elevation. Unfortunately, the proportion of elderly depressed patients who fall into each of these categories is not known. An initial positive response was observed in 46 of 71 (65%) depressed inpatients of average age 71.8 years who were administered a single 20-mg oral dose of methylphenidate; in another study, variable dosages of methylphenidate (up to 30 mg per day over a 5-day period) were administered to a somewhat younger group of depressed patients, and the rate of positive response was 60%.

COMBINATION THERAPY

Several combinations of medications have been claimed to be effective for depression resistant to single-drug treatment. These include:

- Benzodiazepine and cyclic or MAOI antidepressant
- MAOI and cyclic antidepressant
- Cyclic antidepressant augmented by thyroid hormone (T_4 or T_3)
- Cyclic antidepressant augmented by estrogen
- Cyclic antidepressant or MAOI augmented by lithium

Controlled studies of these combinations in elderly patients per se are lacking, and the available general psychopharmacologic literature is equivocal at best regarding the antidepressant efficacy of any except lithium augmentation, which has been shown in several controlled studies to convert 25–50% of tricyclic antidepressant nonresponders to responders in 5–15 days. Case reports and our clinical experience with elderly patients indicate similar efficacy in nonresponders to trazodone and MAOIs as well, although controlled studies with these agents are lacking.

The following procedure is recommended: after a 3- to 4-

week trial of antidepressant at maximum tolerable dosages (supported by determination of adequate serum levels where appropriate; see above), lithium is added in low doses and titrated to acute treatment levels, i.e., 0.8–1.2 meq/ml. Generally, side effects are additive, although the above-described clinical experience raises the possibility that gross intention/action tremor may follow the particular combination of lithium and fluoxetine. Rapid response (i.e., within 3–5 days) is common, but some patients require up to 2 weeks of augmentation before peak response occurs. We have treated several patients who responded dramatically within the first 24–48 hours and then deteriorated to prelithium status within another few days; formal reports describing this early response–early escape phenomenon have yet to be published.

With respect to the other drug combinations listed, little can be said in favor of MAOI and cyclic antidepressant, cyclic antidepressant and thyroid hormone, or cyclic antidepressant and estrogen; however, combining a benzodiazepine with a cyclic or MAOI antidepressant, although not providing greater antidepressant effect per se, may be useful for control of anxiety and agitation in the first few weeks of therapy. This can be particularly beneficial when nonsedating agents such as fluoxetine, protriptyline, and tranylcypromine are prescribed. Dosages are as for each agent prescribed alone.

■ TREATMENT OF PSYCHOTIC DEPRESSION

Although geriatric depression accompanied by hallucinations and/or delusions is relatively refractory to psychopharmacologic therapy, acceptable remission can often be obtained with the combination of antipsychotic agents and antidepressants. Psychotic symptoms are treated with high-potency, low-dose agents such as haloperidol before initiating antidepressant therapy. The end point of antipsychotic treatment is not eradication of symptoms, which may require several months of treatment, but control of the affective and behavioral consequences of psychosis. When fear, social withdrawal, attempts to hide or otherwise protect oneself from fantasized persecutors, sleeplessness, and hypervigilance are reduced, delusions and hallucinations may be described as "empty," even though delusional content may continue to be articulated with apparent conviction, and hallucinations may continue to be reported. At this point, which typically requires several days of antipsychotic treatment, antidepressants may be prescribed and titrated to therapeutic dosage levels with little risk of exacerbating psychosis.

■ ELECTROCONVULSIVE THERAPY

Electroconvulsive therapy (ECT) remains the single most effective treatment for major depression with or without psychosis in elderly patients. Remission rates in the 90%+ range are typical, and side effects are usually limited to transient memory impairment. Although ECT is approximately equally effective in psychotic and nonpsychotic depression, the relatively limited effectiveness of psychopharmacologic therapy in the former condition makes psychotic depression the strongest indication for ECT as a first-line therapy. Other indications for ECT as the treatment of first choice include:

- Active suicidality
- High likelihood of inability to tolerate antidepressant side effects
- High likelihood of medication noncompliance

Perhaps the most common indication for ECT, however, is psychopharmacologic treatment failure.

Unilateral, nondominant electrode placement minimizes memory impairment, but the literature to date and our clinical experience raise a serious question about the comparative efficacy of unilateral treatment, particularly when the newer brief-pulse machine is used.

An effective approach is to use brief-pulse, bilateral electrode placement, administering three treatments per week. The switch to unilateral placement is made only if memory impairment threatens to endanger the patient or causes sufficient subjective distress to threaten continued compliance with treatment. Psychopharmacologic treatments other than benzodiazepine anxiolytics and hypnotics and low-dose haloperidol as needed for anxiety, sleep, agitation, or psychosis are discontinued during the course of ECT, and routine pretreatment anticholinergics are not prescribed. Seizures are monitored using the cuff-isolation technique, and stimuli producing a seizure of less than 25 seconds duration are repeated.

Treatments are administered until symptom reduction has reached a plateau and three treatments have been administered on the plateau. This approach requires an average of 11 treatments to produce full remission. Prophylactic antidepressant treatment is initiated immediately after the last treatment.

The associated anterograde memory impairment, which is cumulative over the course of treatment, typically reaches the level of mild disorientation to time and mild recent-memory loss. Both of these symptoms usually clear rapidly and are clinically undetectable in a few days, although occasionally they persist for as many as 3 or 4 weeks. Retrograde memory loss, especially for events occurring during the course of treatment, may persist much longer, and memory for some intrahospitalization events may be permanently lost. Given this information, along with the above recovery statistics and the extremely low mortality rate of ECT (less than one death per 10,000 cases), the great majority of patients are readily willing to accept this degree of memory loss as part of the "cost" of treatment. As is clear from the above discussion, there are many important factors to consider in the treatment of major depression in the elderly. To avoid repetition and redundancy, treatment should be systematic and logical. Figure 4-1 presents one useful flow diagram for this therapy.

■ TREATMENT OF BIPOLAR DISORDER

PSYCHOSOCIAL TREATMENT

Psychosocial treatment of mania and hypomania is typically oriented toward optimizing compliance with somatic therapies and assisting patients and families with the often daunting task of establishing and maintaining appropriate behavioral boundaries. Counseling and support are often also useful in the aftermath of a hypomanic or manic episode, when patients may find themselves alienated from friends, family, treating physicians, and other

84

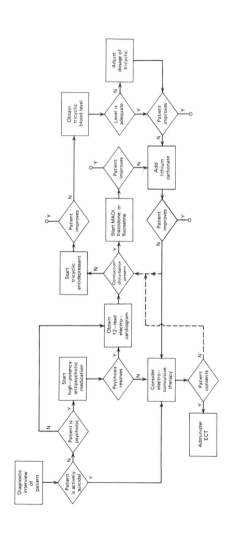

FIGURE 4-1. **Flow diagram for treatment of major depression.**
ECT = electroconvulsive therapy. MAOI = monoamine oxidase inhibitor.

caretakers. Generally, insight-oriented therapies are avoided during the acute phase of illness, but may be quite effective when the most severe symptoms are under control. Both individual and family-therapy approaches can be used, whereas group settings may not provide enough structure to allow the hypomanic or manic elderly patient to benefit.

SOMATIC TREATMENT

Psychopharmacologic management of hypomania or mania in the older patient is usually a two-phase process: the first phase aims at establishing rapid control of symptoms, followed by the second phase in which the goals are subacute control of symptoms and long-term prophylaxis. Pretreatment evaluation was described earlier.

Perhaps the most widely used strategy for the first phase begins with administration of high-potency, low-dose neuroleptic medications such as haloperidol, fluphenazine, or thiothixene, either orally or by intramuscular injection. Doses are gradually increased (from 1 to 40 mg per day for haloperidol and fluphenazine, double that for thiothixene) as needed to control symptoms. Once symptoms are controlled, oral administration of lithium carbonate is initiated with small doses (e.g., 150 mg twice per day). After 3–5 days, the plasma lithium level is determined, and lithium dosages are titrated to achieve a plasma level in the 0.6–1.0 meq/ml range. Finally, gradual tapering of the neuroleptic is undertaken. Potential side effects (and their management) include those associated with neuroleptic medications (see Chapter 6) and lithium (see above) as well as acute confusion that can progress to frank delirium, apparently induced by a lithium-neuroleptic interaction. Each of these side effects is reversible and usually responds to dosage reduction.

In this strategy, dosages of neuroleptic may be minimized by adjunctive administration of oral or intramuscular lorazepam, 0.25–1.0 mg every 4–6 hours as needed; however, caution is recommended with this combination because the occasional patient may "paradoxically" react to lorazepam with increased disinhibition. Dosages of lithium required for long-term prophylaxis are typically lower than those appropriate for middle-aged adults, and plasma levels may also be lower; otherwise, principles of management are essentially the same as for younger patients.

LONG-TERM LITHIUM MANAGEMENT

As is the case for young adults, prophylactic plasma levels are generally lower than those required for acute symptom reduction, typically in the 0.3–0.8 meq/ml range. Although it is true that elderly patients are somewhat more prone to develop toxicity at relatively low plasma levels, management is guided by clinical response, and multiple plasma level determinations are rarely useful or necessary.

OTHER MOOD-STABILIZING AGENTS

Carbamazepine is the most thoroughly studied mood-stabilizing agent besides lithium and has been shown to have acute antimanic effects and to provide effective long-term prophylaxis in patients with bipolar disorder. Although there are no studies in the elderly per se, available data suggest that carbamazepine may be most effective in manic patients who cycle rapidly and who have predominantly irritable rather than euphoric mood. As mentioned above, these features have been reported to occur commonly in elderly manic patients, suggesting that carbamazepine may have a relatively greater role in the elderly than in middle-aged and young patients. At present, however, carbamazepine is mainly used as an anticonvulsant and is reserved for use in bipolar patients unresponsive to lithium. Dosages (typically beginning at 200 mg po twice a day) are titrated to produce blood levels in the 4–12 μg/ml range, and antimanic effects take 4–7 days to appear.

Side effects and adverse reactions from carbamazepine include sedation, dizziness, ataxia, nausea and vomiting, mild anticholinergic effects, skin rash (rarely including Stevens-Johnson syndrome and toxic epidermal necrolysis), and worsening of congestive heart failure, hypertension, and hypotension. Rare cases of aplastic anemia and agranulocytosis have also been reported, necessitating baseline blood studies and periodic repeat evaluations. Although data indicating increased sensitivity to these side effects and adverse reactions in older patients have not been published, carbamazepine is metabolized in the liver and the general pharmacokinetic and pharmacodynamic considerations discussed in Chapter 2 apply.

Other anticonvulsants reported to have antimanic effects include sodium valproate and clonazepam. Experience with the former in elderly patients is limited, and solid recommendations remain to be articulated. Clonazepam is discussed in Chapter 6.

■ REFERENCES

1. Spar JE: Principles of diagnosis and treatment in geriatric psychiatry, in Essentials of Geriatric Psychiatry. Edited by Lazarus LW. New York, Springer, 1988, pp 102–113

2. Thompson LW, Gallagher D, Breckenridge JS: Comparative effectiveness of psychotherapies for depressed elders. J Consult Clin Psychol 55:385–390, 1987

3. Steuer J, Mintz J, Hammen CL, et al: Cognitive-behavioral and psychodynamic group psychotherapy in treatment of geriatric depression. J Consult Clin Psychol 52:180–189, 1984

4. Gerson SC, Plotkin DA, Jarvik LF: Antidepressant drug studies 1964 to 1986: empirical evidence for aging patients. J Clin Psychopharmacol 8:311–322, 1988

5. Nelson JC, Jatlow P, Quinlan DM, et al: Desipramine plasma concentration and antidepressant response. Arch Gen Psychiatry 39:1419–1422, 1982

6. Kutcher SP, Shulman KI, Reed K: Desipramine plasma concentration and therapeutic response in elderly depressives: a naturalistic pilot study. Can J Psychiatry 31:752–754, 1986

7. Kutcher SP, Reid K, Dubbin JD, et al: Electrocardiogram changes and therapeutic desipramine and 2-hydroxy-desipramine concentrations in elderly depressive patients. Br J Psychiatry 148:676–679, 1986

8. Schneider LS, Cooper TB, Staples FR, et al: Prediction of individual dosage of nortriptyline in depressed elderly outpatients. J Clin Psychopharmacol 7:311–314, 1987

9. Spar JE: Plasma trazodone concentrations in elderly depressed inpatients: cardiac effects and short-term efficacy. J Clin Psychopharmacol 7:406–409, 1987

10. Spar JE, LaRue A: Major depression in the elderly: DSM-III criteria and the dexamethasone suppression test as predictors of treatment response. Am J Psychiatry 140:844–847, 1983

11. Jarvik LF, Read SL, Mintz J, et al: Pretreatment orthostatic hypotension in geriatric depression: predictor of response to imipramine and

doxepin. J Clin Psychopharmacol 3:368–372, 1983

12. Schneider LS, Sloane RB, Staples FR, et al: Pretreatment orthostatic hypotension as a predictor of response to nortriptyline in geriatric depression. J Clin Psychopharmacol 6:172–176, 1986

13. Spar JE, LaRue A: Acute response to methylphenidate as a predictor of outcome of tricyclic antidepressant therapy in the elderly. J Clin Psychiatry 46:466–469, 1985

14. Bernstein J: Drug Therapy in Psychiatry. Boston, John Wright, 1983

15. Georgotas A, McCue RE, Hapworth W, et al: Comparative efficacy and safety of MAOIs versus TCAs in treating depression in the elderly. Biol Psychiatry 21:1155–1166, 1986

6 DEMENTIA AND DELIRIUM

■ GENERAL DIAGNOSTIC CONSIDERATIONS

APPROACH TO THE PATIENT

HISTORY

An accurate history of the present illness is particularly important in the diagnostic evaluation of dementia, because it can establish the temporal relationships between possible organic etiologies and the onset of cognitive decline, help to differentiate primary degenerative from multi-infarct dementia, and permit the potentially important distinction between early- and late-onset Alzheimer's disease. Accordingly, multiple sources of information, including past medical records, should be used to supplement information provided by the patient and the patient's primary caregiver, and an attempt should be made to establish detailed timelines. It is particularly important to focus on trauma, signs or symptoms of neurologic or psychiatric illness, substance use including alcohol and medications, and past and present exposure to potential toxins, as well as past surgeries and past and present psychosocial stressors. The family history should include inquiry about Down's syndrome, dementia, and neurological or mental illness.

MENTAL STATUS EXAMINATION

A comprehensive clinical mental status examination remains the cornerstone of the diagnosis of dementia. General categories of appearance; level of alertness; degree of cooperation; mood; affect (direction and degree); form, flow, and content of thought; psychomotor activity; presence or absence of hallucinations, delusions, and other morbid thought content; and judgment and insight are assessed along with cognitive function.

DEMENTIA RATING SCALES

Assessment of cognitive function on clinical mental status examination may be supplemented by administration of a structured mental status examination of the type described below. Results of these procedures can provide a valuable baseline for assessing treatment-related cognitive changes and can also be used to determine if a referral for neuropsychological assessment is desirable or feasible.

There are many different cognitive mental status examinations available, and several, including the Information-Memory-Concentration Test (1), the Mini-Mental State Exam (MMSE) (2), and the Mattis Dementia Rating Scale (3) have been extensively used with geriatric patients.

Table 5-1 lists major sections and sample items from the Mattis Dementia Rating Scale, which is the most comprehensive of the mental status instruments developed for older adults. Items are hierarchically arranged within sections, so that the first item serves as a screen for intact ability in each domain. The Mattis Dementia Rating Scale provides more extensive assessment of language, memory, and praxis than most mental status examinations and includes items that may be sensitive to frontal lobe impairment (initiation and perseveration sections). Although a normal elderly person can complete this test in 10–15 minutes, 30–45 minutes may be required for patients with cognitive problems. The cutoff score for screening for dementia is 123 or fewer correct out of a possible 144. This scale is recommended for use with mildly impaired patients, when a detailed assessment of

TABLE 5-1. **Overview of Mattis Dementia Rating Scale**

Cognitive function tested	Sample items
Attention	Digit span; responds to 2 successive commands
Initiation and perseveration	Verbal: name things to buy at supermarket; name articles of clothing; repeat words, sounds
	Motor: imitate alternating hand movements; copy alternating patterns
Construction	Copy complex or simple figures
Conceptualization	Similarities; name things people eat, wear, ride; identify word that doesn't fit in group; identify figure that doesn't fit in group
Memory	Recall examiner's sentence; generate and recall own sentence; recognition memory for words, designs

Source: Adapted from Mattis S: Mental status examination for organic mental syndrome in the elderly patient, in Geriatric Psychiatry. Edited by Bellak L, Karasu TB. New York, Grune & Stratton, 1976, pp 77–121.

abilities is desired, and when time permits complete administration.

Figures 5-1 and 5-2 display items from the widely used MMSE, which is a 30-point scale based on 11 items tapping orientation, concentration, memory, language, and motor skills. The MMSE was initially validated with several elderly psychiatric groups and normal community control subjects and has been included in several independent validation studies. It has been found to have high interrater reliability and adequate retest reliability in stable conditions. The usual recommended cutoff score for cognitive impairment is 23 or fewer correct. Folstein and colleagues have emphasized that the MMSE does not establish a diagnosis of dementia; instead, it identifies individuals with possible cognitive impairment that may warrant further assessment. Although sensitivity and specificity of the MMSE are adequate for most screening applications, caution should be exercised in interpreting low scores in poorly educated individuals. Also, the MMSE may fail to detect focal brain impairment if interpretation is limited to the total-correct score.

Table 5-2 presents a third, and very brief, mental status examination, the Orientation-Memory-Concentration Test (4). This is a derivative of the Information-Memory-Concentration Test developed by Blessed et al. (1). One point is scored for each incorrect response and then multiplied by the weighting factor given in Table 5-2; the maximum total weighted error score is 24, and scores of 10 or greater are considered consistent with dementia. This test is not recommended for use with mildly impaired individuals or those who may only have focal deficits. However, it can be useful in serial assessment of patients with known dementia or in situations where large numbers of older people must be efficiently screened.

RATINGS OF EVERYDAY BEHAVIOR

Several brief rating scales have been developed for use with family members or other caregivers to identify problems in everyday functioning. The Blessed Dementia Index (Table 5-3) (1) consists of 22 items evaluating basic activities of daily living (e.g., ability to shop, manage money, and find one's way around) and personality and behavior change (e.g., increased rigidity, diminished emotional responsiveness, purposeless hyperactivity). Severity of impairment on this scale has been shown to correlate significantly with neuropathologic changes of Alzheimer's disease.

Another widely used functional scale is the Instrumental Activities of Daily Living Measure developed by Lawton and Brody (5), which consists of eight items assessing areas of function considered crucial for maintaining independent living in the community (e.g., using the telephone, shopping, responsibility for medications). Including one of these measures in the diagnostic workup of patients with cognitive impairment can help to clarify the severity of everyday dysfunction and can identify areas of need for supportive services.

During the mental status examination, it is important to establish rapport, reduce anxiety, and eliminate external distracters, so as to obtain the patient's best possible performance

Patient _____

Examiner _____

Date _____

Maxi-mum score	Score	
		Orientation
5	( )	What is the (year) (season) (date) (day) (month)? Where are we? (state) (country) (town) (hospital) (floor)
		Registration
3	( )	Name 3 objects: 1 second to say each. Then ask the patient all 3 after you have said them. Give 1 point for each correct answer. Then repeat them until he or she learns all 3. Count trials and record. Trials _____
		Attention and Calculation
5	( )	Serial 7s. One point for each correct. Stop after 5 answers. Alternatively spell "world" backward.
		Recall
3	( )	Ask for the 3 objects repeated above. Give 1 point for each correct.

Language

9   ( )   Name a pencil, and a watch (2 points).
Repeat the following "No ifs, ands, or buts" (1 point).
Follow a 3-stage command:
    "Take a paper in your right hand, fold it in half, and put it on the floor" (3 points)
Read and obey the following:

Close your eyes (1 point)

Write a sentence (1 point)
Copy design (1 point)

Total score
ASSESS level of consciousness
  along a continuum

Alert	Drowsy	Stupor	Coma

FIGURE 5-1.   **Mini-Mental State Exam.** Adapted from Folstein MF, Folstein SE, McHugh PR: "Mini-Mental State": a practical method for grading the cognitive state of patients for the clinician. J Psychiatr Res 12:189–198, 1975.

Orientation

(1) Ask for the date. Then ask specifically for parts omitted, e.g., "Can you also tell me what season it is?" One point for each correct.

(2) Ask in turn "Can you tell me the name of this hospital?" (town, country, etc.). One point for each correct.

Registration

Ask the patient if you may test his or her memory. Then say the same of 3 unrelated objects, clearly and slowly, about 1 second for each. After you have said all 3, ask the patient to repeat them. This first repetition determines score (0–3) but keep saying them until he or she can repeat all 3, up to 6 trials. If he or she does not eventually learn all 3, recall cannot be meaningfully tested.

Attention and Calculation

Ask the patient to begin with 100 and count backward by 7. Stop after 5 subtractions (93, 86, 79, 72, 65). Score the total number of correct answers.

If the patient cannot or will not perform this task, ask him or her to spell the word "world" backward. The score is the number of letters in correct order, e.g., dlrow = 5, dlorw = 3.

Recall

Ask the patient if he or she can recall the 3 words you previously asked him or her to remember. Score 0–3.

Language

Naming: Show the patient a wrist watch and ask him or her what it is. Repeat for pencil. Score 0–2.

Repetition: Ask the patient to repeat the sentence after you. Allow only one trial. Score 0 or 1.

3-Stage command: Give the patient a piece of plain blank paper and repeat the command. Score 1 point for each part correctly executed.

Reading: On a blank piece of paper print the sentence "Close your eyes," in letters large enough for the patient to see clearly. Ask him or her to read it and do what it says. Score 1 point only if the patient actually closes his or her eyes.

Writing: Give the patient a blank piece of paper and ask him or her to write a sentence for you. Do not dictate a sentence; it is to be written spontaneously. It must contain a subject and a verb and be sensible. Correct grammar and punctuation are not necessary.

Copying: On a clean piece of paper, draw intersecting pentagons, each side about 1 inch, and ask the patient to copy it exactly as it is. All 10 angles must be present, and 2 must intersect to score 1 point. Tremor and rotation are ignored. Estimate the patient's level of consciousness along a continuum, from alert on the left to coma on the right.

FIGURE 5-2. **Instructions for administration of Mini-Mental State Exam.** Adapted from Folstein MF, Folstein SE, McHugh PR: "Mini-Mental State": a practical method for grading the cognitive state of patients for the clinician. J Psychiatr Res 12:189–198, 1975.

TABLE 5-2. The six-item Orientation-Memory-Concentration Test

Item	Maximum error	Score	Weight
What year is it now?	1	X	4 =
What month is it now?	1	X	3 =
Repeat this phrase after me: John Brown, 42 Market Street, Chicago			
About what time is it?	1	X	3 =
Count backward from 20 to 1	2	X	2 =
Say the months in reverse order	2	X	2 =
Repeat the memory phrase	5	X	2 =

Source: Adapted from Katzman R, Brown T, Fuld P, et al: Validation of a short orientation-memory-concentration test of cognitive impairment. Am J Psychiatry 140:734–739, 1983.

and minimize deficits related to lack of concentration, cooperation, or effort.

LABORATORY EVALUATION

Laboratory evaluation is aimed at identifying illnesses known to cause dementia and generally begins with a selected standardized battery of tests with relatively high sensitivity and low specificity. The screening battery in Table 5-4 was recommended by a National Institutes of Health Consensus Development Conference in 1987 (6).

The following additional procedures may be of value depending on clinical circumstances:

- *Computed tomography* (CT). This procedure is valuable to rule out mass lesion such as tumor or subdural hematoma and may help to identify normal-pressure hydrocephalus.
- *Magnetic resonance imaging* (MRI). MRI may be more sensitive than CT for identification of ischemia, infarction, and subcortical and brain stem pathology. Otherwise, the two procedures have a similar role in the evaluation of dementia.

TABLE 5-3. **Blessed Dementia Index**

Changes in performance of everyday activities:

1. Inability to perform household tasks, e.g., cooking, maintenance (0,½,1) [a]
2. Inability to handle small sums of money (0,½,1)
3. Inability to remember short lists of items, e.g., in shopping (0,½,1)
4. Inability to find way about indoors (0,½,1)
5. Inability to find way about familiar streets (0,½,1)
6. Inability to interpret surroundings (e.g., to recognize whether in hospital or at home; to discriminate between patients, doctors, and nurses) (0,½,1)
7. Inability to recall recent events (e.g., recent outings, visits of relatives and hospital staff) (0,½,1)
8. Tendency to dwell in the past (0,½,1)
9. Eating: cleanly, with proper utensils (0); messily, with spoon only (1); with fingers only (2); has to be fed (3)
10. Dressing: unaided (0); occasionally misplaced buttons, etc. (1); wrong sequence, commonly forgetting items (2); unable to dress (3)
11. Continence: complete sphincter control (0); occasional urinary incontinence (1); frequent urinary incontinence (2); doubly incontinent (3)

Changes in personality and habits:

12. Increased rigidity (0,1) [b]
13. Increased egocentricity (0,1)
14. Impairment of regard for feelings of others (0,1)
15. Coarsening of affect (crude, unrefined expression of emotion) (0,1)
16. Impairment of emotional control (e.g., increased petulance and irritability) (0,1)
17. Hilarity in inappropriate situations (0,1)
18. Diminished emotional responsiveness (0,1)
19. Sexual misdemeanor (appearing de novo in old age) (0,1)
20. Hobbies, pastimes, interests relinquished (0,1)
21. Diminished initiative or growing apathy (0,1)
22. Purposeless hyperactivity (0,1)

TOTAL SCORE _____

[a] Scoring options (in parentheses): 0 = no change; ½ = partial, variable, or intermittent incapacity; 1 = complete incapacity.
[b] 0 = no change; 1 = change.
Source. Adapted from Blessed G, Tomlinson B, Roth M: The association between quantitative measures of dementia and of senile change in the cerebral grey matter of elderly subjects. Br J Psychiatry 114:797–811, 1968.

TABLE 5-4. **Laboratory evaluation of dementia**

Routine studies	Special studies
• Complete blood count • Electrolyte panel • Screening metabolic panel • Thyroid function tests • Vitamin B_{12} and folate levels • Tests for syphilis • Tests for human immunodeficiency antibodies, as indicated by history • Urinalysis • Electrocardiogram • Chest X ray	• Computed tomography (CT) of head—to rule out mass lesion, normal-pressure hydrocephalus • Magnetic resonance imaging of head—same indications as for CT, may be more sensitive for ischemia or infarction, subcortical or brain stem pathology • Electroencephalogram (EEG)—to evaluate ictal or episodic features of history or mental status examination; preliminary data suggest a possible wider role for computerized topographic EEG (7) • Lumbar puncture—to rule out central nervous system infection suggested by physical examination

- *Electroencephalogram* (EEG). EEG is indicated when episodic or ictal features are present in the history or mental status examination, or if intoxication is suspected and cannot be otherwise demonstrated. Preliminary research suggests a possible role for the computerized EEG, particularly as applied to topographic data (7).
- *Lumbar puncture.* This is indicated when other findings (e.g., nuchal rigidity, unexplained elevation of white blood cell count or fever) point to possible infection of the central nervous system.

NEUROPSYCHOLOGICAL TESTS

Neuropsychological tests are often ordered to corroborate an impression of dementia and to identify specific cognitive strengths and weaknesses that may have a bearing on treatment or placement recommendations. Table 5-5 summarizes some of the tests that we have found useful in diagnostic assessment for possible dementia. Each of these tests has been developed for geriatric applications or has been studied extensively with older patients. Other measures may be useful as well, but any battery to be used in dementia evaluation should tap a full range of cognitive abilities, including general intelligence, attention, language, learning and memory, visuospatial performance, and reasoning or problem solving. If there are questions of coexisting psychiatric disturbance, psychodiagnostic measures should also be included (see Chapter 4).

Neuropsychological testing alone is not generally sufficient to establish a particular etiology for dementia. However, the pattern of performance on these tests can either strengthen or weaken the case for certain types of dementia. For example, on tests of learning and memory, reduced recall relative to age, combined with frequent errors of intrusion, perseveration, or confabulation, are commonly observed in dementia of the Alzheimer type, but are less often noted in subcortical dementias (e.g., Huntington's chorea or Parkinson's disease) or in major depression.

■ SECONDARY DEMENTIA

DIAGNOSTIC EVALUATION

In a minority of patients with dementia, there is "evidence from the history, physical examination, or laboratory tests of a specific organic factor (or factors) judged to be etiologically related to the disturbance" (8, p. 107). In patients in whom these organic factors primarily affect extracerebral tissues and only secondarily lead to "brain failure," the term *secondary dementia* has been applied. Secondary dementias are, at least in some patients, preventable, arrestable, or reversible, if the underlying illness is diagnosed and treated before significant brain damage has occurred.

The prevalence of secondary dementia is quite variable, with reported frequencies ranging from 5 to 58%, depending on the

TABLE 5-5. **Examples of neuropsychological assessment instruments**

Test	Description	Functions assessed	Interpretation	Comment
Wechsler Adult Intelligence Scale—Revised (WAIS-R) [a]	General adult intelligence battery with 11 subtests; normed to age 75	Verbal and nonverbal skills including vocabulary, attention, reasoning, visuoconstruction, and perceptual-motor integration	Age-corrected subtest scores ≤7 may indicate impairment	Influenced by education
Wechsler Memory Scale—Revised (WMS-R) [b]	Battery of verbal and nonverbal memory tests; normed to age 75	Orientation, mental control, memory span, immediate and delayed recall of stories, designs, and word pairs	Memory quotient <85 or low subscale percentile rankings may indicate impairment	Sensitive to mild amnesia, dementia
Selective Reminding Test [a]	Memorization of a list of 12 words;	Short-term and long-term memory;	Recall of ≤50% or absence of learning	May help to distinguish memory

	provisional norms for elderly patients	retrieval; ability to benefit from reminders	curve suggests impairment	deficits of dementia vs. depression
Boston Naming Test [a]	Naming of drawings of objects; normed to ages 80+	Confrontation naming, access to semantic knowledge	Cutoff scores vary with age, education	Sensitive to mild anomic aphasia that may not be detected in mental status testing
Controlled Word Association Test [a]	Naming of words beginning with specified letters; age and education norms	Verbal fluency, access to semantic memory	Cutoff scores vary with age, education	Repetitions, intrusion, noted in early Alzheimer-type dementia
Trail Making Test [a]	Lines drawn to connect number and letter sequences; provisional norms to ages 80+	Composite index of visual scanning, sequencing, mental flexibility, visuomotor integration	Cutoff scores vary with age	Failure on alternating sequence often noted on mild brain injury

For references to tests, see [a] Lezak M: Neuropsychological Assessment, 2nd Edition. New York, Oxford University Press, 1983; [b] Wechsler D: Wechsler Memory Scales—Revised. New York, Psychological Corporation, 1986.

population sampled. Although the determinants of this prevalence have not been clearly identified, socioeconomic factors, including the availability and quality of medical care in the sampled community, are likely to be important.

COMMON ETIOLOGIES

Among the most frequently reported causes of secondary dementia are normal-pressure hydrocephalus, brain tumor, endocrinopathy (especially hypothyroidism), and medications, especially those with central anticholinergic effects. In general, the list of organic etiologies capable of causing dementia increases with the age of the patient, as declining functional brain reserve reduces the individual's ability to tolerate physiologic derangement. In the frail elderly, disorders as innocuous as urinary tract infection can indirectly lead to cognitive impairment severe enough to warrant a diagnosis of dementia. Table 5-6 lists common organic causes of dementia.

MANAGEMENT

Management of patients with suspected secondary dementia entails diagnostic evaluation followed by specific therapy aimed at correcting or arresting the organic factor responsible for the dementia. Oral and parenteral administration of deficient vitamins, surgical correction of normal-pressure hydrocephalus and brain tumor, thyroid hormone replacement, or discontinuation of anticholinergic medications may all result in restoration of lost cognitive function or halt progression in patients in whom irreversible brain damage has already occurred. Residual behavioral and mood symptoms may then be treated following the principles discussed later in this chapter under "Psychopharmacologic Treatment of Alzheimer's Disease."

■ PRIMARY DEMENTIA

The primary dementias reflect organic pathology of the brain that, unchecked, invariably leads to intellectual deterioration. About 60% of all primary dementias are associated with brain

TABLE 5-6. **Organic factors that can cause dementia**

Infections
- Acquired immunodeficiency syndrome
- Creutzfeldt-Jakob disease
- Cryptococcosis
- Leptomeningitis, encephalitis
- Progressive multifocal leukoencephalopathy
- Syphilis
- Whipple's disease

Intoxications
- Medications
- Antihypertensives
- Corticosteroids
- Digitalis
- Opiates and synthetic narcotics
  Psychoactive agents with anticholinergic properties
  Other chemicals
  Carbon disulfide, carbon monoxide
  Lead, manganese, mercury
  Most drugs of abuse

Metabolic disorders
- Dehydration
- Diabetes
- Pulmonary disease with hypoxia or hypercarbia
- Renal, hepatic failure
- Thyroid, parathyroid, adrenal, or pituitary disease

Neurological disorders
- Alzheimer's disease
- Amyotrophic lateral sclerosis
- Cerebellar and spinocerebellar degeneration
- Huntington's chorea
- Multiple-system atrophy
- Normal-pressure hydrocephalus
- Olivopontocerebellar degeneration
- Parkinson's dementia complex of Guam
- Parkinson's disease
- Progressive subcortical gliosis
- Progressive supranuclear palsy

TABLE 5-6. **Organic factors that can cause dementia**
(continued)

Nutritional disorders
- Folate deficiency
- Pellagra
- Pernicious anemia
- Thiamine deficiency

Space-occupying lesions
- Brain tumor
- Chronic subdural hematoma
- Obstructive hydrocephalus

Vascular disorders
- Atherosclerosis, arteriosclerosis
- Hypertension
- Repeated episodes of cerebral ischemia or hypoxia
- Vasculitis

neuropathology of the Alzheimer type, another 15–20% with multiple brain infarctions, and about 15–20% with both conditions simultaneously; the remaining 10% are attributable to rare conditions, including Creutzfeldt-Jakob disease and end-stage Huntington's chorea.

ALZHEIMER'S DEMENTIA

Alzheimer's disease, including both early-onset (onset before age 65) and late-onset subtypes, accounts for about 60% of all cases of primary dementia. Because the diagnosis of Alzheimer's disease requires visualization of characteristic neuropathology (i.e., senile plaques and neurofibrillary tangles) in brain tissue of affected patients, Alzheimer's disease is at best a "probable" diagnosis in the living patient. In DSM-III-R, the term *primary degenerative dementia of the Alzheimer type* is applied to patients who meet clinical and laboratory criteria for probable Alzheimer's disease; however, because even the most carefully selected series may include cases of Pick's disease or other primary dementing diseases, the terms *Alzheimer's disease* and *primary degenerative dementia of the Alzheimer type* are not absolutely interchangeable. Because of this inherent diagnostic uncertainty, epidemiologic data on the prevalence of Alzheimer's disease per se contain an irreducible element of unreliability; still, multiple surveys converge on a prevalence of Alzheimer's dementia at about the 5–6% range in the population over age 65 and indicate that within this group, the prevalence climbs steeply to about 20% of individuals in their 80s.

In the remainder of this section, the term *Alzheimer's disease* will be used to refer to primary degenerative dementia of the Alzheimer type, of presenile or senile onset, unless otherwise specified.

CLINICAL PRESENTATION

As is true for all dementing illnesses, the clinical presentation of Alzheimer's disease depends on the stage of illness and may be complicated by symptoms related to concomitant physical and psychiatric illness, including depressed mood, anxiety, suspiciousness, and psychosis. Table 5-7 summarizes the clinical and laboratory findings typically observed as the disease progresses (9).

HISTORY

The history of Alzheimer's disease is typically one of insidious onset and gradual progression of cognitive impairment, with few of the sharp downward steps in function typical of multi-infarct dementia, or the more abrupt onset and rapid progression of the dementia syndrome of depression. Some cognitive deficits can be covered or compensated for, and friends and family who have only superficial interactions with patients may be unaware of major deficits; close family members who have observed declining function may attempt to rationalize away the significance of their observations. Because of these possibilities, multiple sources of historical data may be necessary to establish a reliable history.

About one-third of patients with Alzheimer's disease suffer psychotic symptoms at some time during the course of their illness (10). In some of these patients, the psychosis is clinically prominent enough to obscure the underlying cognitive impairment and delay accurate diagnosis. Delusions are usually per-

106

TABLE 5-7. **Natural history of Alzheimer's disease: clinical findings**

Function/ test	Early cognitive decline	Moderate cognitive decline	Severe cognitive decline
Orientation	Fully oriented	Frequent mistakes but usually knows date, familiar persons	Severe disorientation
Concentration	Mild deficits, some errors in serial calculations	Moderate deficits; usually has difficulty counting backward	Can barely count to 10
Recent memory	Misplaces items; forgets names, recent events	Poor knowledge of current and recent events	Unaware of almost all recent experiences
Remote memory	Some deficits in recall of remote events	Many deficits in recall of remote events	Almost no recall of any past events
Language/ speech	Word-finding problems, poor word-list generation, mild anomia	Limited vocabulary and sentence structure, repetitive	Fluent aphasia with unintelligible speech
Praxis	Normal to minimal deficits	Ideomotor apraxia; difficulty with finances, marketing, hobbies	Cannot feed or toilet self
Visuospatial skills	May get lost in unfamiliar settings; poor constructions on tests	Poor constructions, and spatial disorientation; can travel to familiar destinations	Agraphia; may have neurological signs

TABLE 5-7. **Natural history of Alzheimer's disease: clinical findings** *(continued)*

Function/ test	Early cognitive decline	Moderate cognitive decline	Severe cognitive decline
Self-care	Normal	May require assistance choosing clothing; may need coaxing to bathe	Requires assistance in all spheres; occasional or persistent incontinence of bladder and bowels
Complex/ new tasks	Decreased performance	Decreased performance; may withdraw from challenging situations	Cannot perform
Personality	Possible depression, apathy, irritability	Denial common; apathy and indifference	Agitation/ anxiety, psychosis, abulia, obsessiveness
CAT scan	Normal	Normal to atrophic cortices and dilated ventricles	Cortical atrophy and ventricular enlargement
EEG	Normal	Background slowing	Diffuse slowing

Source. Adapted with permission from Group for the Advancement of Psychiatry. The Psychiatric Treatment of Alzheimer's Disease. New York, Brunner/Mazel, 1988.

secutory in nature and are typically fragmented and inconsistent, unlike those seen in the common functional disorders (e.g., schizophrenia, delusional disorder, or mood disorder with psychosis). Common delusional content includes the belief that one is being threatened, deprived, or abused by caretakers or that possessions are being stolen. The elaborate "connectedness" seen in functional delusions (i.e., the myriad ways in which the patient is able to tie the delusional belief to all aspects of his or her experience) is usually not present. Similarly, hallucinations, which are usually auditory but can be visual, olfactory, or tactile, are intermittent and of varying, usually trivial content, lacking the ordered, meaningful quality typical of functional hallucinations. Depressed mood as an isolated symptom is also a common accompaniment of Alzheimer's disease, occurring in 40–50% of patients at some time in the course of illness, usually in the earlier stages. Depressive disorders have been reported in only 10–20%, although the range of reported frequency of depressive disorders is large, and this remains a somewhat controversial area of investigation.

MENTAL STATUS EXAMINATION

Some of the major mental status findings typical of each stage of Alzheimer's disease are included in Table 5-7. Although relatively synchronous decline in cognitive capacities is the general rule, in some patients, language disturbance may be severe enough to prevent accurate evaluation of memory and higher cognitive functions; similarly, suspiciousness or social withdrawal may lead to an exaggerated estimate of the degree of cognitive decline in a relatively intact individual.

PATHOGENESIS

Neuropathology

The gross neuropathology of Alzheimer's disease consists of cortical atrophy, particularly involving anterior frontal and temporoparietal areas. Microscopic findings include neurofibrillary tangles, which are densely packed microfibrils found in the cytoplasm of dead neurons. Under an electron microscope, these microfibrils have been shown to consist of paired helical filaments that are 100 angstroms wide and twist every 800 angstroms. They are composed of an unusual protein, with an amino acid composition that has not yet been completely determined. Senile plaques are extracellular deposits 5–150 microns in diameter, consisting of a cluster of fragments of dendrite and axon terminals surrounding a granular core that, in the "classic" plaque, is composed of amyloid. In addition to this classic form, "primitive" forms that lack an amyloid core and "burned out" forms in which the core only is present have also been described (11).

Neurofibrillary tangles and senile plaques are found in greatest density in the frontoparietal and hippocampal cortex and amygdala. Granulovacuolar degeneration affects primarily hippocampal pyramidal neurons and consists of groups of intracytoplasmic vacuoles about 5 microns in diameter, each containing a small granule. Other histopathological findings include congophilic angiopathy, consisting of deposits of amyloid in the walls of small arteries of the frontal and parietal cortex, and generalized loss of neuronal dendrites in affected cortical areas. Loss of cholinergic neurons of the nucleus basalis (nucleus of Meynert) and noradrenergic neurons of the locus coeruleus has also been described and has been correlated with reduced tissue levels of choline acetyltransferase (CAT) and norepinephrine and its metabolites, respectively, as discussed below.

Neurobiochemistry

The first, and most thoroughly confirmed, neurobiochemical abnormality found in brain tissue affected by Alzheimer neuropathology was reduced temporoparietal and hippocampal cortical activity of CAT, an enzyme found only in cholinergic cells that catalyzes the synthesis of acetylcholine. Biopsy studies have demonstrated significant losses of this enzyme as early as the first symptomatic year, and autopsy studies have demonstrated a strong correlation ($r = .8$) between the degree of CAT loss and premortem measurements of cognitive and functional decline. Acetylcholinesterase and acetylcholine, both of which are less specific indicators of cholinergic cell activity, have also been found to be reduced in concentration in affected brain tissue. Altogether, these findings support a working analogy between Alzheimer's disease and Parkinson's disease, in which a single neurotransmitter (dopamine) is also involved. Whereas this analogy initially suggested promising therapeutic approaches and generated much enthusiasm among researchers, the picture has since become significantly more complex as abnormalities in other neurotransmitter systems have been discovered. Table 5-8 summarizes these neurotransmitter findings (12).

TABLE 5-8. **Presynaptic cortical transmitter activities in Alzheimer's disease**

System	Parameter	Status in Alzheimer's disease
Cholinergic	• Choline acetyltransferase	• Consistently reported reduced throughout cortex
	• Acetylcholinesterase	• Dramatic loss histochemically; biochemically extensive loss of tetrameric (G_4) form
	• High-affinity choline uptake	• Decreased
	• Acetylcholine synthesis	• Decreased (biopsy prisms)
Noradrenergic	• Norepinephrine	• Moderate reductions in some areas
	• 3-Methoxy-4-hydroxyphenyl-glycoaldehyde	• Decreased/normal
	• Dopamine β-hydroxylase	• Decreased/normal
Dopaminergic	• Dopamine	• Near normal
	• Homovanillic acid	• Near normal
	• Serotonin	• Moderate reductions in some areas
	• 5-Hydroxyindoleacetic acid	• Moderate reductions in some areas
γ-Aminobutyric acid (GABA)	• GABA	• Normal
	• Glutamate decarboxylase	• Normal in biopsy (decreased in autopsy tissue)
	• K^+-evoked GABA release	• Normal in biopsy prisms
Glutamic (and aspartic) acid	• Free amino acid	• Normal
	• K^+-evoked release	• Normal in biopsy prisms
Somatostatin	• Neuropeptide immunoreactivity	• Reduced

TABLE 5-8. **Presynaptic cortical transmitter activities in Alzheimer's disease** (continued)

System	Parameter	Status in Alzheimer's disease
Corticotropin-releasing factor	• Neuropeptide immunoreactivity	• Reduced
Substance P Met-enkephalin Neuropeptide Y Cholecystokinin Vasoactive intestinal polypeptide Neurotensin Thyrotropin-releasing hormone	• Neuropeptide immunoreactivity	• Generally normal

Source. Adapted from Perry EK: Cortical neurotransmitter chemistry in Alzheimer's disease, in Psychopharmacology: The Third Generation of Progress. Edited by Meltzer HY. New York, Raven, 1987, p 889. With permission. Copyright 1987 Raven Press, Ltd.

Genetics

There is fairly wide agreement among investigators that genetic factors are involved in the pathogenesis of Alzheimer's disease. Observations that support this view include:

- Patients with Down's syndrome (trisomy 21) invariably develop the histopathological hallmarks of Alzheimer's disease if they live into their 40s, and the prevalence of Down's syndrome in families of patients with Alzheimer's disease is increased over that seen in the general population.
- Over 50 pedigrees of families have now been reported in which Alzheimer's disease is transmitted as an apparent autosomal dominant gene. Although these families represent only a small fraction of all cases, they raise the question of whether a similar gene is operating in so-called sporadic cases of Alzheimer's disease.
- The largest family study in which all probands had autopsy-confirmed Alzheimer's disease found a 45% cumulative risk of disease by age 84 in siblings of probands who had an affected

parent and became symptomatic before age 70 (13). Rates of occurrence of Alzheimer's disease in probands' and family members' spouses, who are presumably subjected to similar environmental influences, did not differ from that of the general population. Similar findings have emerged from studies in which probands were diagnosed by clinical criteria only. Although the interpretation of Heston et al.'s (13) data as evidence for an autosomal dominant Alzheimer's gene has been challenged by subsequent studies, they comprise strong evidence for a genetic influence of some type.

Two major problems confront investigators in this area:

- The apparent variability of age at expression of the Alzheimer gene(s), as illustrated by one report of identical twins discordant for the disease for at least 20 years after the onset of illness in the affected twin (14). This variability must result in some "genotypic" patients with Alzheimer's disease dying before the gene can be expressed.
- The requirement that diagnoses of Alzheimer's disease probands be confirmed by autopsy study implies that family studies that do not do so are likely to include phenocopies (cases in which a non-Alzheimer's genotype mimics phenotypical Alzheimer's disease). Death of genotypic family members before their disease is apparent and inclusion of phenocopies both result in underestimates of the influence of genetic factors in the pathogenesis of disease.

Taking all data together, perhaps the hypothesis for which most support has been collected at present is that Alzheimer's disease occurs when genetic influences result in increased susceptibility to an environmental factor or factors, such as those discussed below.

Other Theories of Etiology

Many other etiologic theories of Alzheimer's disease have been advanced, including brain tissue hypoperfusion secondary to atherosclerosis or sludging of blood in cerebral capillaries, aluminum intoxication, uncomplicated aging, viral infection, and autoimmune mechanisms. Obviously, these theories are not all logically equivalent; all but viral infection could be conceptualized as pathogenetic mechanisms in search of an etiology. Little evidence has been adduced for hypoperfusion; the fact that 80% of octogenarians are free of Alzheimer's disease effectively rules out normal aging per se, and the lack of a correlation between exposure to aluminum and rates of illness seems to militate against aluminum intoxication. The notion that a viral infection could cause Alzheimer's disease was initially suggested by the existence of so-called slow-virus (e.g., scrapie) infections in animals, which share several features with Alzheimer's disease; i.e., they are slowly progressive, involve the central nervous system, and at least in some instances appear late in the animal's life span. Unfortunately, scores of attempts to transmit Alzheimer's disease to animal hosts have failed, and the viral theory has accordingly lost much of its earlier appeal.

Evidence in support of autoimmune mechanisms has been similarly indirect. The presence of amyloid in senile plaques and in the walls of arterioles was an early hint that autoimmune mechanisms may be involved, but subsequent studies of humoral and cellular immune function, brain reactive antibodies, and the major histocompatibility complex in patients with Alzheimer's disease generally have failed to provide strong evidence of immune system involvement in the etiology or pathogenesis of Alzheimer's disease. However, recent research demonstrating a common protein subunit known as amyloid-beta-protein in senile plaque amyloid, arterial amyloid, and neurofibrillary tangle protein (15) has rekindled interest in this area of investigation.

DIAGNOSIS

The diagnosis of Alzheimer's disease requires the patient to meet criteria for dementia and a history of insidious onset and gradual progression; if all other causes of dementia are ruled out by the history, physical examination, and laboratory tests, the diagnosis of dementia of the Alzheimer type is made (see Table 5-9).

NINCDS Criteria

The National Institute of Neurological and Communicative Disorders and Stroke (NINCDS) recently published a set of diagnos-

TABLE 5-9. **Diagnostic criteria for dementia and primary degenerative dementia of the Alzheimer type**

Diagnostic Criteria for Dementia

A. Demonstrable evidence of impairment in short- and long-term memory.

B. At least one of the following:
   (1) Impairment in abstract thinking
   (2) Impaired judgment
   (3) Other disturbances of higher cortical function, such as aphasia, apraxia, agnosia, and "constructional difficulty"
   (4) Personality change, i.e., alteration or accentuation of premorbid traits

C. The disturbance in A and B significantly interferes with work or usual social activities or relationships with others.

D. Not occurring exclusively during the course of delirium.

E. Either (1) or (2):
   (1) There is evidence of a specific organic factor (or factors) judged to be etiologically related to the disturbance, or
   (2) In the absence of such evidence, an etiologic organic factor can be presumed if the disturbance cannot be accounted for by any nonorganic mental disorder.

Diagnostic Criteria for Primary Degenerative Dementia of the Alzheimer Type

A. Dementia (see above)
B. Insidious onset with a progressive deteriorating course
C. Exclusion of all other causes of dementia by history, physical examination, and laboratory tests

Source. Adapted with permission from American Psychiatric Association: Diagnostic and Statistical Manual of Mental Disorders, 3rd Edition, Revised. Washington, DC, American Psychiatric Association, 1987, pp 107, 121. Copyright 1987 The American Psychiatric Association.

tic criteria for research purposes that are somewhat more narrow than DSM-III-R criteria (16). Separate standards are listed for the clinical diagnosis of probable versus possible Alzheimer's disease (see Table 5-10).

TABLE 5-10. **Criteria for clinical diagnosis of Alzheimer's disease (AD) from the National Institute of Neurological and Communicative Disorders and Stroke—Alzheimer's Disease and Related Disorders Association work group**

I. Criteria for PROBABLE AD:
_____ Dementia
_____ Established by clinical examination
_____ Documented by MMSE, Blessed Dementia Index or similar examination
_____ Confirmed by neuropsychiatric testing
_____ Deficits in >2 areas of cognition
_____ Progressive loss of memory *and* cognitive functions
_____ No disturbance of consciousness
_____ Onset between ages 40 and 90
_____ Absence of systemic disorders or other brain diseases that in and of themselves could account for deficits

II. Diagnosis of PROBABLE AD supported by:
_____ Progressive loss of specific cognitive functions (e.g., language, motor skills, perception)
_____ Impaired ADLs and altered behavior patterns
_____ Family history of similar disorders, especially if neuropathologically confirmed
_____ Lab results of
_____ Normal lumbar puncture
_____ Normal or nonspecific changes on EEG
_____ CT—cerebral atrophy with progression documented by serial observation

III. Other features consistent with PROBABLE AD:
_____ Plateaus in course of progression of illness
_____ Associated symptoms (e.g., depression, incontinence, weight loss)
_____ Seizures in advanced disease
_____ CT normal for age

IV. PROBABLE AD uncertain if:
_____ Sudden onset
_____ Focal neurological findings
_____ Seizures or gait disturbance early in course of illness

TABLE 5-10. **Criteria for clinical diagnosis of Alzheimer's disease (AD) from the National Institute of Neurological and Communicative Disorders and Stroke—Alzheimer's Disease and Related Disorders Association work group**
(continued)

V. POSSIBLE AD:

_____Dementia syndrome in absence of other causes and in presence of *variations* in onset, presentation, or clinical course of

_____A second systemic or brain disorder sufficient to produce dementia but not considered *the* cause

_____*Single*, gradually progressive severe cognitive deficit

VI. DEFINITE AD:

_____Clinical criteria for PROBABLE AD with neuropathological confirmation

VII. Subtypes

_____Familial

_____Onset before age 65

_____Presence of trisomy 21

_____Other relevant disorders (e.g., parkinsonism)

Note. MMSE = Mini-Mental State Exam. ADLs = activities of daily living. CT = computed tomography.
Source. Adapted with permission from McKhann G, Drachman D, Folstein M, et al: Clinical diagnosis and Alzheimer's disease: report of the NINCDS-ADRDA work group under the auspices of Department of Health and Human Services Task Force on Alzheimer's Disease. Neurology 34:939–944, 1984.

Laboratory Evaluation

Laboratory evaluation of Alzheimer's disease is the same as described above for dementia (Table 5-4). Despite some promising work described later in this chapter, there are as yet no laboratory test results specific for Alzheimer's disease, and the laboratory evaluation is primarily aimed at ruling out other causes of dementia.

Neuropsychological Tests

In probable Alzheimer's disease, multiple neuropsychological impairments are present, including anomic or mixed aphasia, apraxia, deficits in reasoning, and prominent learning and memory impairment. Patients with Alzheimer's disease often do not benefit from cuing or memory reminders, implying deficits in encoding or learning as well as problems with retrieval. Early in the course of illness, neuropsychological deficits may be restricted to one or two areas, most often learning and memory.

Experimental Diagnostics

As above, research in several areas has included computer-analyzed EEG (CEEG), positron emission tomography (PET), single photon emission computer tomography (SPECT), cerebrospinal fluid antigens, monoclonal antibodies to paired helical filaments and plaque protein, recombinant DNA investigation of genetic markers (particularly on chromosome 21), and others, but, as yet, there are no diagnostic tests that significantly improve the approximately 90% accuracy (i.e., 10% false-positive rate as determined at autopsy) that can be obtained with DSM-III-R and NINCDS clinical criteria.

Differential Diagnosis

Other dementias. The differential diagnosis of Alzheimer's disease includes the functional conditions that can mimic dementia (mainly depressive pseudodementia [see Chapter 4]; more rarely, mania, hypomania, personality disorder, Ganser syndrome, hysteria, and malingering) and the secondary and primary dementias (Table 5-6). For practical purposes, the major alternative possibility on statistical grounds, after secondary and functional causes have been ruled out, is multi-infarct dementia, which can generally be ruled out using scales such as the Hachinski, as described below.

Rare conditions such as Creutzfeldt-Jakob disease can usually be identified by characteristic clinical features like myoclonus, seizures, and a very rapidly progressive course, as well as by typical changes on the clinical EEG. Pick's disease may be identified by a characteristic pattern of cortical atrophy (as demonstrated by CT or MRI), in which there is relative sparing of parietal cortex, and correspondingly relative absence of aphasia and apraxia. In some cases of Pick's disease, only frontal cortex is affected, and symptoms are correspondingly limited to personality change, with little memory impairment.

Alcoholic dementia and the subcortical dementias can usually be differentiated from Alzheimer's dementia by the presence of a strong history of alcohol ingestion and relative sparing of constructional ability in the former, and the characteristic disorders of movement in the latter. The typical features of these dementing illnesses are described below.

Amnestic syndromes. These can be mistaken for dementia, even though in amnestic syndrome intellectual functions other than memory are spared. The most common amnestic syndrome in elderly patients is likely to be Korsakoff's psychosis, which is caused by prolonged thiamine deficiency usually associated with chronic high-dose ingestion of alcohol. Besides sparing of intellect, confabulation is often a prominent feature of this syndrome.

Delirium. Alzheimer's disease is usually easily differentiated from delirium, which has a much more acute onset and progression and entails more severe impairment of attention and concentration and more disorganization of thought. However, delirium superimposed on Alzheimer's disease may be more difficult to diagnose, often requiring reevaluation after potential causes of delirium have been eliminated and the underlying dementia has been allowed to emerge.

Functional disorders. As described above, many functional disorders can present with dementia that at least superficially resembles Alzheimer's disease. In the majority of patients, the signs and symptoms of functional illness are clear, cognitive impairment is readily identified as secondary, and diagnostic error is easily avoided. Still, some cases are quite misleading, and several authorities have recommended antidepressant treatment trials in questionable cases (see Figure 4-1 and related discussion, Chapter 4).

TREATMENT

Psychosocial

The role of individual psychotherapy in the overall medical management of the patient with Alzheimer's disease depends on the stage of illness, the patient's premorbid pattern of ego strengths and vulnerabilities, and the presence or absence of concomitant functional complications. In general, supportive therapy is most useful in the early stages of illness and is aimed at ameliorating the anxiety and loss of self-esteem accompanying awareness and anticipation of lost cognitive capabilities. Many patients at this stage of illness use primitive defenses including denial, projection, somatization, and displacement, resulting in characteristic symptom complexes: accusations that family members are stealing from them (denial and projection), hypercritical and hostile behavior directed toward family members (denial and displacement), and multiple, sometimes bizarre somatic complaints (somatization). For some of these patients, the capacity for insight is preserved, and gentle interpretation may lead to adaptive behavior change, particularly if accompanied by practical advice and encouragement. Later in the course of illness, individual psychotherapy has more limited goals, often limited to provision of a constant, caring, healing authority figure whose attention can have significant, if nonspecific, anxiety-relieving and mood-elevating effects (9).

Behavioral approaches, ranging from operant conditioning to group experiences aimed at remotivation and reality orientation, have been of limited value in patients with Alzheimer's disease, probably because of the limited capacity for learning common to those patients impaired enough to be candidates for these techniques. The Group for the Advancement of Psychiatry report (9) and a book edited by Jarvik and Winograd (17) contain reviews of this literature.

Family intervention is useful at all stages of illness (18, 19). Initially, key elements of family therapy include dissemination of practical advice, information and education, referral to appropriate community resources, and provision of an opportunity to ventilate emotions and express fears related to the diagnosis. Later, family therapy may be more focused on amelioration of caregiver anxiety, demoralization, and depression. In the final stages of illness, consultation and support vis-à-vis the often painful decision to institutionalize, and assistance with the process of grieving a "lost" loved one, may become the foci of family therapy.

Psychopharmacological Treatment of Alzheimer's Disease

Neuroleptics. Perhaps the most common, and most debilitating, symptom complex seen in patients with Alzheimer's disease is agitation, which is often accompanied by paranoid ideation with or without hallucinations, belligerent and hostile behavior, and physical aggressiveness. Agitation, which may occur in acute, discrete episodes or as a subacute or chronic state, is a syndrome of pathological arousal typically manifested as repetitive, compulsive motor activity (e.g., pacing, picking at clothes, social intrusiveness), accompanied by impaired attention and concentration; elevated heart rate and blood pressure, tremor, and tachypnea may also be seen in agitated patients. Verbalizations may range from reasonably articulate if perseverative expressions of apprehension and fear to pressured incoherence, screaming, and cursing. Although all agitated patients are anxious, agitation as described herein rarely remits completely with anxiolytic agents alone, except in occasional mild instances (see below).

Neuroleptics comprise one phase of a two-phase treatment approach. First, the patient and the patient's physical and social environment are examined to determine what, if any, reversible factors are contributing to the agitation. Circumstances in which patients feel discomfort and are unable (usually because of cognitive impairment) to take corrective action can lead to agitation. Accordingly, simple interventions such as helping the patient to the bathroom, correcting underlying congestive heart failure or urinary tract infection, or providing reorientation or reassurance are often effective. After these measures have been undertaken, residual symptoms of agitation can be treated with neuroleptic medications, preferably of the high-potency, low-dose type. Haloperidol, fluphenazine, and thiothixene are among the agents in this category that have proven to be most useful. Typical dosages range from 0.5 to 5 mg of haloperidol (or equipotent dosages of fluphenazine or thiothixene), administered orally or by intramuscular injection for acute agitation; if repeated episodes occur, or agitation becomes chronic, initiation of a daily regimen in the same dose range is usually effective. At these dosages, extrapyramidal side effects (i.e., akinesia, rigidity, and tremor) are rarely a serious problem, and other side effects of these agents are generally negligible.

Lower-potency, higher-dose agents such as thioridazine are generally avoided because of their greater anticholinergic potency, which can increase confusion in patients with Alzheimer's disease, and their propensity to cause other side effects such as orthostatic hypotension. The high-potency agents are likewise effective when agitation is accompanied by hallucinations, belligerent and hostile behavior, or physical aggressiveness. If these symptoms fail to respond to neuroleptic therapy at dosages low enough to avoid significant extrapyramidal side effects, augmentation with lorazepam, 0.5–1 mg administered orally or by intramuscular injection, is usually effective. A typical daily regimen could include a standing order for 2 mg of haloperidol orally at bedtime, and 0.5 mg of lorazepam orally every 4–6 hours, either as a standing order or as needed.

Anxiolytics. Although not as disruptive as the agitation syndrome, patients with Alzheimer's disease are also susceptible to anxiety in various forms and degrees of severity. Although treatment with anxiolytics is generally guided by the same principles that apply to the nondemented elderly (see Chapter 7), patients with Alzheimer's disease may be unable to articulate subjective feelings of apprehension, psychomotor tension, or fear, and the clinician often must rely on more objective signs. In this regard, mild agitation as described above can reflect an anxiety state and may respond to anxiolytics alone.

Antidepressants. Although authorities disagree on the prevalence of clinical depressive disorders in patients with Alzheimer's disease, it is clear that such disorders do occur and can be quite disabling, often leading to increased cognitive impairment (a syndrome that has been termed "pseudopseudodementia"). The principles that guide treatment of depression in the nondemented elderly (see Chapter 4) apply, with the following modifications:

- Tricyclic agents and others with central anticholinergic potency are avoided when possible because patients with Alzheimer's disease, by virtue of cholinergic system disruption, are particularly susceptible to adverse reactions ranging from subtle worsening of cognitive function to frank delirium. Accordingly, monoamine oxidase inhibitors (in circumstances in which medications and diet can be adequately monitored), trazodone, and fluoxetine are felt by many to be the treatments of first choice.

- Patients with Alzheimer's disease may not be able to articulate subjective feelings of sadness, hopelessness, helplessness, or worthlessness, and the clinician must rely on neurovegetative signs and nonverbal expressions of mood as target symptoms for treatment. The latter may include refusal to eat, crying spells, facial expressions of sadness or pain, unexplained episodes of agitation or hostility, and increased confusion.
- Patients with Alzheimer's disease may similarly not describe subjective side effects of medications, such as postural lightheadedness or dizziness, so routine measurements of orthostatic blood pressure and careful assessment of gait and balance may be somewhat more necessary than in the nondemented elderly patient.

Other agents. Lithium, carbamazepine, and other mood-stabilizing agents may be prescribed for patients with Alzheimer's disease with bipolar mood disorder or its variants, with considerations as above. Benzodiazepine hypnotic agents are prescribed as for the nondemented elderly. The common practice of prescribing diphenhydramine and other antihistamines as hypnotics is particularly inadvisable for patients with Alzheimer's disease because these agents have significant anticholinergic potency and can cause increased cognitive impairment. Psychostimulants such as methylphenidate have a minor role in treatment of patients with Alzheimer's disease. Although it has been repeatedly demonstrated that these agents do not improve cognitive function, they can be effective for apathy and social withdrawal and are occasionally useful to reverse sedative side effects of other agents.

Experimental approaches. The literature on experimental treatments of Alzheimer's disease is too vast to be summarized here, but several excellent review articles are listed at the end of the chapter. In general, psychostimulants, anticoagulants, vasoactive peptides, aluminum chelating agents, so-called nootropic agents (e.g., piracetam, centrophenoxine, vincamine), vasodilators, narcotic antagonists, and acetylcholine precursors have been shown to be ineffective in arresting or reversing cognitive impairment in patients with Alzheimer's disease. On the other hand, acetylcholine-enhancing agents such as physostigmine (a cholinesterase inhibitor) and arecoline, an acetylcholine agonist, have been shown to produce minor, clinically insignificant improvement in some measures of memory and higher cognitive function. Similarly, dihydrogenated ergot alkaloids, originally believed to have vasodilating effects but now known primarily to affect the metabolism of glucose in brain tissue, have also been shown to produce mild improvement in global functioning in patients with early Alzheimer's disease. The mechanism of this action is not known, and specific efficacy vis-à-vis cognitive functions per se has yet to be conclusively demonstrated; some investigators have speculated that the efficacy of dihydrogenated ergot alkaloids may be due to mild antidepressant or psychostimulating properties.

Two recent developments in experimental treatment of Alzheimer's disease warrant special mention here. Tetrahydroaminoacridine (THA) was reported in one well-publicized study to produce "dramatic" improvement in several patients with Alzheimer's disease (20), and a large-scale multicenter study designed to test this claim is underway at the time of this writing. However, the original study employed questionable methodology, and subsequent investigation by the Food and Drug Administration has raised doubt about some of the data reported in the article. Accordingly, great optimism does not seem warranted in anticipation of the outcome of the multicenter study.

Intracerebral infusion of bethanechol has been attempted by several centers, using an abdominally implanted pump to deliver medication directly into the cerebral ventricles (21). To date, no group data have been published indicating efficacy of this approach, but informal accounts of occasional subjects (perhaps those with more "pure" cholinergic system disease) who function better on active drug than on placebo (administered according to a double-blind protocol) seem to warrant "cautious expectation" in this area of investigation.

MULTI-INFARCT DEMENTIA

EPIDEMIOLOGY

The prevalence of multi-infarct dementia (MID) per se is not known, but autopsy studies suggest that about 15% of patients with primary dementia have multiple infarctions without histopathological evidence of Alzheimer's disease.

CLINICAL PRESENTATION AND MENTAL STATUS EXAMINATION

Patients with MID present with dementia that may be clinically indistinguishable from other secondary or primary dementias. Presumably because of the episodic nature of the underlying pathophysiology (acute thrombi and/or emboli), the history is typically one of "stepwise progression," with each downward step in function assumed to reflect a new ischemic event. A history (or the presence of) hypertension also strongly correlates with MID, and there may also be a history of transient ischemic attacks or gross infarction. Because of the inherently "patchy" nature of the pathology, mental status examination may reveal mental functions to be affected in an equally "patchy" fashion, with relatively well-preserved islands of function alongside relatively deteriorated areas of function. For example, severe disturbance of language and praxis may coexist with relatively well-preserved memory, or moderate memory impairment may coexist with relative preservation of calculating ability and capacity for abstract thought. Fluctuations in the level of cognitive impairment (e.g., "sundowning") are also reported to be relatively common.

Neurologic examination may reveal focal neurologic signs and symptoms ranging from subtle reflex changes to the pseudobulbar state, particularly if the patient is examined relatively soon after an ischemic event; evidence of systemic atherosclerosis (e.g., peripheral bruits or myocardial infarction) likewise increases the probability of MID.

As is the case with Alzheimer's disease, psychosis may be the presenting problem, and the distinguishing features as described above generally apply to MID as well as to Alzheimer's disease.

PATHOGENESIS

MID is believed to be caused by the cumulative effects on brain function of multiple small cortical and subcortical infarctions. Although generalized arteriosclerosis secondary to hypertension, cerebral atherosclerosis, and diabetes are usually cited as the most common causes of thrombotic infarction, and cardiac disease and carotid atherosclerosis as the most common causes of embolic infarction, Cummings and Benson (22) list over 70 distinct conditions that can lead to MID. Within the category of MID, several subtypes (e.g., lacunar state, Binswanger's disease, granular atrophy) have been distinguished on the basis of the specific location of infarctions, but there is little evidence that these subtypes have any particular clinical or epidemiological significance.

DIAGNOSIS

DSM-III-R criteria for MID are displayed in Table 5-11. A rating scale (23) (Table 5-12) designed to quantify the probability of underlying infarctions in the demented patient has been published based on the clinical signs and symptoms described above. Unfortunately, this scale cannot rule out concomitant degenerative diseases such as Alzheimer's disease, which occurs in about 50% of patients with autopsy-proven multiple infarctions. Liston and LaRue (24,25) have published a detailed critique of the logic,

TABLE 5-11. **Diagnostic criteria for multi-infarct dementia**

A. Dementia (see p. 107 of DSM-III-R)

B. Stepwise deteriorating course with "patchy" distribution of deficits (i.e., affecting some functions, but not others) early in the course

C. Focal neurologic signs and symptoms (e.g., exaggeration of deep tendon reflexes, extensor plantar response, pseudobulbar palsy, gait abnormalities, weakness of an extremity).

D. Evidence from history, physical examination, or laboratory tests of significant cerebrovascular disease (recorded on Axis III) that is judged to be etiologically related to the disturbance.

Source. Adapted with permission from American Psychiatric Association: Diagnostic and Statistical Manual of Mental Disorders, 3rd Edition, Revised. Washington, DC, American Psychiatric Association, 1987, p 123. Copyright 1987 The American Psychiatric Association.

TABLE 5-12. **Clinical features of the Modified Ischemic Score**

Feature	Point values
Abrupt onset	2
Stepwise deterioration	1
Somatic complaints	1
Emotional incontinence	1
History or presence of hypertension	1
History of strokes	2
Focal neurologic symptoms	2
Focal neurologic signs	2

Note. A score of 4 or more is consistent with multi-infarct dementia.
Source. Adapted from Rosen WG, Terry RD, Fuld PA, et al: Pathological verification of ischemic score in differentiation of dementias. Ann Neurol 7:486–488, 1980.

methodology, and clinical and pathological data on which DSM-III-R criteria for MID and the Rosen et al. (23) scale are based.

Laboratory Evaluation

Laboratory evaluation when MID is suspected is the same as that described above for dementia. The laboratory evaluation is aimed at ruling out secondary dementias and accumulating direct and indirect evidence for multiple cerebral infarctions. Brain imaging procedures such as CT or MRI may directly demonstrate multiple infarctions, in which case diagnostic confidence is clearly increased; on the other hand, infarctions may be too small to be picked up by these procedures, and a negative scan cannot be interpreted as ruling out MID.

Neuropsychological Tests

Because MID can result from many different cerebrovascular conditions, neuropsychological findings are variable. Many MID patients exhibit deficits suggesting subcortical impairment, including pronounced psychomotor slowing, depression, difficulty retrieving learned information, and mild frontal deficits (e.g., reduced ability to plan actions, problems shifting attention from one task to another). On tests of learning and memory, MID patients may benefit considerably from cues and may have normal recognition memory. Other MID patients demonstrate subcortical and cortical neuropsychological pathology.

Differential Diagnosis

Other dementias. As is the case with all of the dementing illnesses, the differential diagnosis of MID includes the secondary dementias, the primary dementias, the subcortical dementias, and functional illness with cognitive impairment.

Delirium. Delirium is generally distinguishable from MID by the much more acute onset and rapid progression seen in delirium, as well as by the nature and severity of cognitive deficits typical of the two conditions. However, the diagnostic picture can be clouded in two situations: when MID and true delirium occur simultaneously and during an episode of acute confusion (e.g., "sundowning") of the type to which MID patients are prone, particularly in the early evening. "Sundowning," which is usually a self-limiting, transient state, may present many of the features of delirium without the implications of deranged physiology and poor prognosis characteristic of true delirium. Accurate diagnosis of MID in both cases depends on reevaluation when signs or symptoms of delirium or acute confusion have cleared, allowing the underlying dementia to be characterized.

Functional disorders. As described above, a number of functional illnesses can mimic dementia of any type, including MID. Generally, these illnesses will be identifiable by the rapid onset and progression of symptoms and the atypical overall clinical picture (i.e., absence of neurological signs and symptoms, hypertension, etc.) seen in the functional disorders.

TREATMENT

As is the case for Alzheimer's disease, there is no specific treatment for MID. Psychosocial and psychopharmacologic therapy follow the general principles outlined above for Alzheimer's disease. Treatment aimed at controlling hypertension and cardiac arrythmia may help prevent further strokes, as may prescription of aspirin or other anti-platelet-aggregating agents.

OTHER DEMENTIAS

SUBCORTICAL DEMENTIA

Several neurological conditions in which the most prominent brain pathology is found in subcortical structures are also associated with dementia, particularly in the late stages of illness. These conditions include parkinsonism and progressive supranuclear palsy, Huntington's chorea, Wilson's disease, some cases of MID, and other rare conditions. The dementia associated with these conditions, according to several authors, includes psychomotor retardation, a type of forgetfulness that has been termed "dilapidation of recall," difficulty with complex problem solving and concept formation, and a relative absence of "cortical" features including aphasia, apraxia, and agnosia. Stooped posture and shuffling gait have also been cited as part of the picture of subcortical dementia. Although debate continues regarding the precise pathophysiology of dementia in the above illnesses, as well as its prevalence and "subcortical purity," dementia as described above clearly occurs in some patients and is a potentially important consideration in the diagnostic process.

ALCOHOLIC DEMENTIA

The precise nosological status of the neuropsychological abnormalities associated with prolonged heavy ingestion of alcohol remains a topic of some debate. Some patients diagnosed with alcoholic dementia are likely suffering from Korsakoff's psychosis, concomitant Alzheimer's disease, or MID or are displaying the effects of continued intoxication (26). Still, the available evidence suggests that substantial cognitive deficits are common in heavy drinkers, and that even though these deficits tend to remit after drinking is discontinued, some deficits may persist for years and may in fact be permanent. Studies using CT have demonstrated significant cortical atrophy and cerebral ventricular enlargement in an unexpectedly large proportion of alcoholic patients (27), even in the absence of clear intellectual impairment, although the precise clinical significance of these findings and the details of the underlying pathology and pathophysiology remain to be elucidated.

RARE CONDITIONS

Dementia occurs in Creutzfeldt-Jakob disease, a rare viral encephalopathy that usually includes myoclonic jerks, seizures, and mixed motor neuron and pyramidal tract signs, in addition to a clinically nonspecific dementia. Acquired immunodeficiency syndrome (AIDS) also causes dementia, apparently by direct viral invasion of brain tissue and by facilitating other central nervous system viruses such as herpes, and a dementia is commonly seen in patients undergoing long-term kidney dialysis. The latter condition has been associated with increased brain and serum levels of aluminum, which is used in the construction of dialysis machines.

■ DELIRIUM

EPIDEMIOLOGY

The prevalence of delirium depends on the population at risk. Liston (28) estimates that 50% or more of elderly patients on psychiatric wards may be delirious at any given time, with those over age 75 at greatest risk.

CLINICAL PRESENTATION

HISTORY

Delirium is a syndrome of cerebral dysfunction of acute or subacute onset that occurs most commonly in patients with significant intra- or extracerebral organic pathology. Accordingly, the medical history is typically that of the primary illness, with a superimposed history of the development of attentional deficits, disorganization of thought, alterations in the level of consciousness, etc., as outlined below. For obvious reasons, the delirious patient usually cannot give a reliable history of the present illness, which is obtained from friends, family, hospital personnel, or the medical record. Because delirium occurs as an emergent complication of several life-threatening illnesses, it is important to move rapidly through the evaluation.

MENTAL STATUS EXAMINATION

As described below, the most prominent features of delirium are impairment of attention and disorganization of thought. More variable features include altered levels of consciousness, psychomotor agitation or retardation, hallucinations and illusions, disorientation, and memory impairment. Unlike uncomplicated dementia, delirium is rarely disguised by the patient's attempts to cover or minimize deficits. More commonly, the delirious patient cannot participate in a thorough mental status examination, and the syndrome is identified indirectly.

As a step toward more objective diagnosis, a 10-item Delirium Rating Scale (29) (see Table 5-13) has recently been developed. Each item is introduced by a brief statement of rationale for its selection and some rough guidelines for differentiation of symptoms produced by different types of disorders (e.g., affective disorders or schizophrenia versus delirium). To date, the Delirium Rating Scale has only been studied with a small number of

TABLE 5-13. **Items rated on the Delirium Rating Scale**

1. Temporal onset of symptoms

2. Perceptual disturbances

3. Hallucination type

4. Delusions

5. Psychomotor behavior

6. Cognitive status during formal testing

7. Physical disorder

8. Sleep-wake cycle disturbance

9. Lability of mood

10. Variability of symptoms

Source. Adapted from Trzepacz PT, Baker RW, Greenhouse J: A symptom rating scale for delirium. Psychiatry Res 23:89–97, 1988.

patients, and further work examining its utility is needed. In the interim, however, it can be used to provide a list of potentially relevant clinical features to evaluate when delirium is suspected.

PATHOGENESIS

The precise mechanism underlying the clinical picture of delirium is not known, although a final common pathway involving central cholinergic neurons that mediate attention and arousal has been postulated. Indirect evidence for this hypothesis includes the fact that cholinergic neurons appear to be the most sensitive to cerebral hypoxia, which is a fairly potent clinical cause of delirium, and the observation that centrally acting anticholinergic drugs can produce a delirium in otherwise intact individuals that can be reversed by cholinergic-enhancing agents. Given that aging is accompanied by reduced central cholinergic tone, and that many elderly patients have compromised cardiovascular and pulmonary functions rendering them susceptible to hypoxia, it is not surprising that age is a major risk factor for the development of delirium.

DIAGNOSIS

DSM-III-R diagnostic criteria for delirium are displayed in Table 5-14.

LABORATORY EVALUATION

Proper evaluation of delirium requires comprehensive medical evaluation, including a complete physical and neurological examination and laboratory tests as needed. In most circumstances, delirium is encountered by psychiatrists in a consultation role, and the physical examination has been performed by nonpsychiatric personnel. Similarly, laboratory evaluation may have been substantially completed before consultation was requested; the battery of tests listed in Table 5-15 is rather broad-spectrum and can usually be narrowed in the actual clinical situation, depending on the differential diagnosis of the primary illness. A recent study identified four independent factors that were strongly associated with the development of delirium in

TABLE 5-14. Diagnostic criteria for delirium

A. Reduced ability to maintain attention to external stimuli and to appropriately shift attention to new external stimuli

B. Disorganized thinking, as indicated by rambling, irrelevant, or incoherent speech.

C. At least two of the following:
    (1) Reduced level of consciousness
    (2) Perceptual disturbances; misinterpretations, illusions, or hallucinations
    (3) Disturbance of sleep-wake cycle with insomnia or daytime sleepiness
    (4) Increased or decreased psychomotor activity
    (5) Disorientation to time, place, or person
    (6) Memory impairment

D. Clinical features develop over a short period of time (usually hours to days) and tend to fluctuate over the course of a day.

E. Either (1) or (2):
    (1) Evidence from the history, physical examination, or laboratory tests of a specific organic factor (or factors) judged to be etiologically related to the disturbance
    (2) In the absence of such evidence, an etiologic organic factor can be presumed if the disturbance cannot be accounted for by any nonorganic mental disorder, e.g., manic episode accounting for agitation and sleep disturbance

Source. Adapted with permission from American Psychiatric Association: Diagnostic and Statistical Manual of Mental Disorders, 3rd Edition, Revised. Washington, DC, American Psychiatric Association, 1987, p 103. Copyright 1987 The American Psychiatric Association.

elderly hospitalized patients (30). In order of strength of association, these were urinary tract infection, serum albumin less than or equal to 3.4 mg/dl, white blood cell count over 11,000, and proteinuria.

DIFFERENTIAL DIAGNOSIS

In addition to the differential diagnosis of the primary illness underlying delirium, the clinician must rule out other psychiatric illnesses that can present with signs and symptoms similar to true delirium. Dementia can mimic delirium, particularly when agita-

TABLE 5-15. **Laboratory evaluation of delirium**

Screening studies
- Blood studies
    Complete blood count
    Creatinine, electrolytes, glucose, liver function tests, thyroid function
       tests
- Chest X ray
- ECG
- EEG
- Urinalysis, including acetone and glucose

Additional studies
- Blood studies
    Arterial blood gases
    Blood cultures
    Serum drug levels (e.g., digoxin, lithium)
    Serum vitamin B_{12} and folate
    Toxic screen for drugs, alcohol, toxins, heavy metals
- Computed tomography scan of the head
- Lumbar puncture
- Magnetic resonance imaging of the brain
- Serial EEGs
- Urine cultures

Source. Adapted with permission from American Psychiatric Association: Treatments of Psychiatric Disorders: A Task Force Report of the American Psychiatric Association, Vol 2. Washington, DC, American Psychiatric Association, 1989, p 807. Copyright 1989 The American Psychiatric Association.

tion, psychosis, or anxiety is superimposed. In these circumstances, the clinical picture of a disorganized, aroused, confused patient with poor attention and concentration is virtually indistinguishable from delirium, and, even with the knowledge that the patient is demented, the clinician is often obliged to conduct a rapid "mini-evaluation" in which potential causes of delirium, particularly medications with central anticholinergic effects and infection, are ruled out. This "pseudodelirium" is usually self-limited and of very brief duration (minutes to hours), is not accompanied by alterations in the level of consciousness, and may be rapidly responsive to simple reassurance or other behavioral intervention. Functional disorders including mania, hypomania, depression, hysteria, and schizophrenia, particularly in the severe manifestations known as manic delirium and catatonic excitement, can also present with a clinical state that can be impossible to distinguish from an organically caused delirium.

TREATMENT

GENERAL

The first priority is to identify emergent, life-threatening causes of delirium and correct them if possible. The most hazardous of these are acute cerebral ischemia or hypoxia; infection of the central nervous system (meningitis, encephalitis, abscess); intracranial hemorrhage or infarction; acute intoxication with central nervous system depressants, stimulants, anticholinergic agents, or combinations thereof; acute withdrawal of alcohol or other central nervous system depressants; hypoglycemia and hyperglycemia with or without ketoacidosis; acid-base or electrolyte imbalance; acute hyperthyroidism (i.e., "thyroid storm"); and hypertensive encephalopathy.

SPECIFIC PHARMACOLOGIC THERAPY

Two of the above categories of delirium call for specific pharmacologic therapy. Withdrawal of alcohol, benzodiazepines, or barbiturates can produce a characteristic delirium ("delirium tremens," in its most severe form) that is rapidly responsive to treatment with any of the three agents. Practically, benzodiazepines are the treatment of choice and are usually administered parenterally until symptoms are under control, at which time the switch to oral administration can be made. Lorazepam is the benzodiazepine with the most reliable absorption after intramuscular injection and has the additional advantages in elderly patients of having no active metabolites and undergoing one-step hepatic metabolism (i.e., conjugation) that is relatively insensitive to the presence of liver disease. Lorazepam may be administered in dosages of 0.5 mg every hour until symptoms are under control; in more acute situations, intravenous administration affords more rapid onset of action.

The second type of delirium responsive to specific therapy is that caused by centrally acting anticholinergic agents. When withdrawal of the offending agent and supportive therapy are ineffective, further amelioration of symptoms can be attained with parenteral administration of physostigmine, a centrally acting cholinesterase inhibitor. The typical dosage is 2 mg administered intramuscularly or by slow intravenous push. Because physostigmine has a duration of action of only about 60 minutes, whereas most anticholinergic agents are somewhat longer acting, repeated doses may be necessary to achieve a clinically stable situation.

NONSPECIFIC PHARMACOLOGIC THERAPY

In most other situations wherein rapid control of symptoms of delirium is desired, the agent of choice is a high-potency neuroleptic agent such as haloperidol. Although haloperidol will rarely completely reverse delirium, it can control agitation and thereby reduce the danger of self-inflicted injury, exhaustion, or disconnection from vital extracorporeal supports and render the patient more cooperative with appropriate diagnostic and therapeutic interventions. Dosages vary as does route of administration depending on the severity of the clinical situation. Intravenous or intramuscular administration of 5–10 mg will often suffice; when symptoms are refractory, augmentation with 0.5 mg of lorazepam is usually very effective. A detailed protocol for use of haloperidol and lorazepam, along with guidelines for addition of hydromorphone to the regimen, is described by Adams (31).

■ REFERENCES

1. Blessed G, Tomlinson B, Roth M: The association between quantitative measures of dementia and of senile change in the cerebral grey matter of elderly subjects. Br J Psychiatry 114:797–811, 1968
2. Folstein MF, Folstein SE, McHugh PR: "Mini-Mental State": a practical method for grading the cognitive state of patients for the clinician. J Psychiatr Res 12:189–198, 1975
3. Mattis S: Mental status examination for organic mental syndrome in the elderly patient, in Geriatric Psychiatry. Edited by Bellak L, Karasu TB. New York, Grune & Stratton, 1976, pp 77–121
4. Katzman R, Brown T, Fuld P, et al: Validation of a short orientation-

memory-concentration test of cognitive impairment. Am J Psychiatry 140:734–739, 1983

5. Lawton MP, Brody E: Assessment of older people: self-maintaining and instrumental activities of daily living. Gerontologist 9:179–186, 1969

6. National Institutes of Health: Differential diagnosis of dementing diseases. Alzheimers Disease and Associated Disorders 2(1):16–28, 1988

7. Leuchter A, Spar JE, Walter DO, et al: Electroencephalographic spectra and coherence in the diagnosis of Alzheimer's type and multi-infarct dementia. Arch Gen Psychiatry 44:993–998, 1987

8. American Psychiatric Association: Diagnostic and Statistical Manual of Mental Disorders, 3rd Edition, Revised. Washington, DC, American Psychiatric Association, 1987

9. Group for the Advancement of Psychiatry: The Psychiatric Treatment of Alzheimer's Disease. New York, Brunner/Mazel, 1988

10. Wragg RE, Jeste DV: Overview of depression and psychosis in Alzheimer's disease. Am J Psychiatry 146:577–587, 1989

11. Wisniewski HM, Terry RD: Re-examination of the pathogenesis of the senile plaque, in Progress in Neuropathology, Vol 2. Edited by Zimmerman HM. New York, Grune & Stratton, 1973, pp 1–26

12. Perry EK: Cortical neurotransmitter chemistry in Alzheimer's disease, in Psychopharmacology: The Third Generation of Progress. Edited by Meltzer HY. New York, Raven, 1987, pp 887–897

13. Heston LL, Mastri AR, Anderson VE, et al: Dementia of the Alzheimer's type. Arch Gen Psychiatry 38:1085–1090, 1981

14. Renvoize EB, Mindham RHS, Stewart M, et al: Identical twins discordant for presenile dementia of the Alzheimer type. Br J Psychiatry 149:509–512, 1986

15. Masters CL, Multhaup G, Simms G, et al: Neuronal origin of intracerebral amyloid: neurofibrillary tangles of Alzheimer disease contain the same protein as the amyloid of plaque cores and blood vessels. EMBO J 4:2757–2763, 1985

16. McKhann G, Drachman D, Folstein M, et al: Clinical diagnosis of Alzheimer's disease: report of the NINCDS-ADRDA work group under the auspices of Department of Health and Human Services Task Force on Alzheimer's Disease. Neurology 34:939–944, 1984

17. Jarvik LF, Winograd CH (eds): Treatments for the Alzheimer Patient: The Long Haul. New York, Springer, 1988

18. Tune LE, Lucas-Blaustein MJ, Rovner BW: Psychosocial interventions, in Treatments for the Alzheimer Patient: The Long Haul. Edited by Jarvik LF, Winograd CH. New York, Springer, 1988, pp 123–137

19. Zarit SH, Orr NK, Zarit JM: The Hidden Victims of Alzheimer's Disease: Families Under Stress. New York, New York University Press, 1985

20. Summers WK, Majovski LV, Marsh GM, et al: Oral tetrahydro-aminoacridine in longterm treatment of senile dementia, Alzheimer type. N Engl J Med 315:1241–1245, 1986

21. Harbaugh RE, Roberts DW, Coombs DW, et al: Preliminary report: intracranial cholinergic drug infusion in patients with Alzheimer's disease. Neurosurgery 15:514–518, 1984

22. Cummings JL, Benson DF: Dementia: A Clinical Approach. Boston, MA, Butterworths, 1983, pp 138–139

23. Rosen WG, Terry RD, Fuld PA, et al: Pathological verification of ischemic score in differentiation of dementias. Ann Neurol 7:486–488, 1980

24. Liston EH, LaRue A: Clinical differentiation of primary degenerative and multi-infarct dementia: a critical review of the evidence, Part I: clinical studies. Biol Psychiatry 18:1451– 1465, 1983

25. Liston EH, LaRue A: Clinical differentiation of primary degenerative and multi-infarct dementia: a critical review of the evidence, Part II: pathological studies. Biol Psychiatry 18:1467–1483, 1983

26. Lishman WA: Organic Psychiatry. Oxford, Blackwell Scientific Publications, 1987, p 517

27. Ron MA, Acker W, Shaw GK, et al: Computerized tomography of the brain in chronic alcoholism: a survey and follow-up study. Brain 105:497–514, 1982

28. Liston EH: Delirium, in Treatments of Psychiatric Disorders: A Task Force Report of the American Psychiatric Association, Vol 2. Washington, DC, American Psychiatric Association, 1989, pp 804–815

29. Trzepacz PT, Baker RW, Greenhouse J: A symptom rating scale for delirium. Psychiatry Res 23:89–97, 1988

30. Levkoff SE, Safran C, Cleary PD, et al: Identification of factors associated with the diagnosis of delirium in elderly hospitalized patients. J Am Geriatr Soc 36:1099–1104, 1988

31. Adams F: Emergency intravenous sedation of the delirious, medically ill patient. J Clin Psychiatry 49 (suppl 12): 22–26, 1988

■ ADDITIONAL READINGS

Cummings JL: Clinical Neuropsychiatry. New York, Grune & Stratton, 1985

Strub RL, Black FW: Neurobehavioral Disorders: A Clinical Approach. Philadelphia, PA, FA Davis, 1988

6 ANXIETY DISORDERS AND LATE-ONSET PSYCHOSIS

■ **ANXIETY DISORDERS**

EPIDEMIOLOGY

Recent epidemiologic data indicate that anxiety disorders are the most common mental illnesses, with a 1-month prevalence of 7.3% in adults of all ages (1). Interestingly, in adults over age 65, the prevalence falls to 5.5%. Within that group, phobic disorders are the most prevalent (4.8%), followed by obsessive-compulsive disorder (0.8%) and panic disorder (0.1%). The prevalence of generalized anxiety disorder was not reported in this survey. Accurate diagnosis of anxiety disorders in elderly patients can be particularly difficult because of the great overlap between symptoms of anxiety disorder and the "organic" anxiety states associated with various physical illnesses and their treatments. Anxiety may also be a prominent part of almost any other Axis I disorder, including adjustment reaction, dementia, mood disorder, or late-onset psychosis.

CLINICAL PRESENTATION

Whether it occurs in reaction to a transient, time-bound situation, or to a permanent or semipermanent life change, or as part of an anxiety disorder or other Axis I disorder, anxiety presents as a subjective state of dysphoric apprehension or expectation, accompanied by varying combinations of the signs and symptoms listed in Table 6-1. Because the present generation of elderly individuals are particularly disinclined to complain of mental distress, it is not uncommon for anxious elderly patients to focus on these associated features rather than on the subjective state per se. Unfortunately, this often misleads the generalist or internist and results in extensive medical evaluation before the correct diagnosis is appreciated. Even after medical illness has been ruled out, the subjective aspects of anxiety in the elderly may require appreciable clinical skill and sensitivity to elicit. Although anxiety is a major component of panic disorder, phobic disorder, and obsessive-compulsive disorder, in these conditions it is usually clinically "upstaged" by panic attacks, phobic behavior, and compulsive behavior, respectively, and may be reported as almost incidental to these symptoms.

SITUATIONAL ANXIETY

Common situations in which elderly patients experience anxiety are much the same as those that affect adults of all ages and include situations conventionally acknowledged to be anxiety provoking, such as a visit to the dentist or doctor or an airplane flight, as well as those that may seem more idiosyncratic, such as being asked simple mental status examination questions, conducting a

TABLE 6-1. Psychomotor and autonomic features of generalized anxiety disorder

Motor tension
- Trembling, twitching, or feeling shaky
- Muscle tension, aches, or soreness
- Restlessness
- Easy fatigability

Autonomic hyperactivity
- Shortness of breath or smothering sensations
- Palpitations or accelerated heart rate (tachycardia)
- Sweating, or cold clammy hands
- Dry mouth
- Dizziness or lightheadedness
- Nausea, diarrhea, or other abdominal distress
- Flushes (hot flashes) or chills
- Frequent urination
- Trouble swallowing or "lump in throat"

Vigilance and scanning
- Feeling keyed up or on edge
- Exaggerated startle response
- Difficulty concentrating or "mind going blank" because of anxiety
- Trouble falling or staying asleep
- Irritability

transaction with an accountant or a bank teller, or being asked to drive an unfamiliar car.

ADJUSTMENT ANXIETY

In elderly persons, adjustment reactions with anxiety may occur during or after periods of obvious personal crisis and in relationship to crises that may not seem particularly stressful to evaluating professionals. For example, a simple move from one apartment to another, even within the same neighborhood, or from one room in a retirement hotel or board-and-care home to another may precipitate significant anxiety. Similarly, development of a new medical illness, even if it is not life threatening or particularly disabling, may precipitate significant anxiety. Other events that commonly elicit adjustment anxiety include divorce or illness in the family, business or financial reversals, marital strife, or even the long-awaited retirement.

PHOBIC ANXIETY

Although the signal feature of phobic disorder (as described below) is excessive or unreasonable fear of a particular situation, symptomatic anxiety of the type described above also occurs in this disorder when the patient anticipates the feared situation or is unable to avoid it (Table 6-2). New onset of phobic symptoms in elderly patients requires thorough clinical investigation, because in some cases, the fear may turn out to be not so unreasonable. For example, older patients may become afraid to join friends for a game of bridge because of a fear of being unable to follow the action, or of having an episode of incontinence, and subsequent investigation by the clinician may reveal for the first time that such mishaps have actually occurred.

OBSESSIVE-COMPULSIVE DISORDER

Late onset of obsessive-compulsive disorder appears to be quite rare, but older patients can have the condition for many years and only seek medical attention when supervening age-related changes or superimposed mood disorder or dementia force them into treatment. In this situation, the likelihood that compulsive rituals have become "ego-syntonic" and are no longer seen as irrational is increased, and the clinician may be required to ex-

TABLE 6-2. **Diagnostic criteria for simple phobia**

A. A persistent fear of an object or situation, other than fear of having a panic attack, or of humiliation or embarrassment in certain social situations.

B. During some phase of the disturbance, exposure to the specific phobic stimulus almost invariably provokes an immediate anxiety response.

C. The object or situation is avoided, or endured with intense anxiety.

D. The fear or the avoidant behavior significantly interferes with the person's normal routine or with usual social activities or relationships with others, or there is marked distress about having the fear.

E. The person recognizes that his or her fear is excessive or unreasonable.

F. The phobic stimulus is unrelated to the content of the obsessions of obsessive-compulsive disorder or the trauma of posttraumatic stress disorder.

Source. Adapted with permission from American Psychiatric Association: Diagnostic and Statistical Manual of Mental Disorders, 3rd Edition, Revised. Washington, DC, American Psychiatric Association, 1987, pp 244–245. Copyright 1987 The American Psychiatric Association.

plore the early history of the disorder to obtain a less misleading picture. Transient outbreaks of obsessive thoughts and compulsive rituals are not uncommon among elderly patients with major depression with or without psychosis. Unfortunately, DSM-III-R (2) diagnostic criteria as displayed in Table 6-3 are not entirely clear as to the nosological status of such symptoms.

PANIC DISORDER

Elderly patients with panic disorder, particularly of late onset, typically present first to their family physician or internist, who is likely to initiate an evaluation for possible myocardial infarction, transient ischemic attack, or other episodic, life-threatening physical illness. It is usually only after several panic attacks accompanied by negative laboratory tests that the primary physician appreciates the correct diagnosis and seeks psychiatric consultation. Patients and family members are often reluctant to accept that something as terrifying as a panic attack can be "mental," and patients may avoid evaluation by the mental health professional because they fear that they are "losing their minds" or "going

TABLE 6-3. **Diagnostic criteria for obsessive-compulsive disorder**

A. Either obsessions or compulsions:

Obsessions: (1), (2), (3), and (4):

(1) Recurrent and persistent ideas, thoughts, impulses, or images that are experienced, at least initially, as intrusive and senseless.

(2) The person attempts to ignore or suppress such thoughts or impulses or to neutralize them with some other thought or action.

(3) The person recognizes that the obsessions are the product of his or her own mind, not imposed from without.

(4) If another Axis I disorder is present, the content of the obsession is unrelated to it.

Compulsions: (1), (2), and (3):

(1) Repetitive, purposeful, and intentional behaviors that are performed in response to an obsession, or according to certain rules or in a stereotyped fashion.

(2) The behavior is designed to neutralize or to prevent discomfort or some dreaded event or situation; however, either the activity is not connected in a realistic way with what it is designed to neutralize or prevent, or it is clearly excessive.

(3) The person recognizes that his or her behavior is excessive or unreasonable.

B. The obsessions or compulsions cause marked distress, are time-consuming (take more than an hour a day), or significantly interfere with the person's normal routine, occupational functioning, or usual social activities or relationships with others.

Source. Adapted with permission from American Psychiatric Association: Diagnostic and Statistical Manual of Mental Disorders, 3rd Edition, Revised. Washington, DC, American Psychiatric Association, 1987, p 247. Copyright 1987 The American Psychiatric Association.

crazy." Again, although the diagnosis of panic disorder depends on the occurrence of panic attacks as described in Table 6-4, significant anticipatory anxiety is often a major component of the syndrome, and it is usually incorrect to assume that successful pharmacologic amelioration of panic attacks is the end of the story. Reassurance, supportive psychotherapy, and behavior treatment may be necessary before anticipatory anxiety is brought under control.

TABLE 6-4. **Diagnostic criteria for panic disorder**

A. At some time during the disturbance, one or more panic attacks have occurred that were *1)* unexpected, and *2)* not triggered by the attention of others.

B. Either four such attacks have occurred within a 4-week period, or one or more attacks have been followed by a period of at least a month of persistent fear of having another attack.

C. At least four of the following symptoms developed during at least one of the attacks:
   (1) Shortness of breath (dyspnea) or smothering sensations
   (2) Dizziness, unsteady feelings, or faintness
   (3) Palpitations or accelerated heart rate (tachycardia)
   (4) Trembling or shaking
   (5) Sweating
   (6) Choking
   (7) Nausea or abdominal distress
   (8) Depersonalization or derealization
   (9) Numbness or tingling sensations (paresthesias)
   (10) Flushes (hot flashes) or chills
   (11) Chest pain or discomfort
   (12) Fear of dying
   (13) Fear of going crazy or of doing something uncontrolled

D. During at least some of the attacks, at least four of the C symptoms developed suddenly and increased in intensity within 10 minutes of the beginning of the first C symptom noticed in the attack.

E. It cannot be established that an organic factor initiated and maintained the disturbance, e.g., amphetamine or caffeine intoxication, hyperthyroidism.

Source. Adapted with permission from American Psychiatric Association: Diagnostic and Statistical Manual of Mental Disorders, 3rd Edition, Revised. Washington, DC, American Psychiatric Association, 1987, pp 237–238. Copyright 1987 The American Psychiatric Association.

PATHOGENESIS

PSYCHODYNAMIC THEORIES

The general psychodynamic literature on the pathogenesis of anxiety is too voluminous to attempt to summarize here, although relatively little consideration has been given to anxiety in late life.

In addition to intrapsychic conflict between the demands of conscience, the limitations imposed by circumstances, and libidinal impulses and emotions, which is postulated to account for anxiety throughout the life span, elderly individuals also face anxiogenic circumstances peculiar to senescence. These include the growing discrepancy between past and present capabilities and the increasing likelihood of incompetence, as well as the reality of death. Anxiety related to these concerns may emerge directly into consciousness, wherein it can be relatively easily identified, or may remain unconscious and be expressed indirectly as somatic dysfunction, memory impairment, or nonspecific illness. In support of this hypothesis, it is often the case that improved emotional well-being is associated with increased conscious awareness of, and ability to, "come to terms with" these aspects of aging.

NEUROBIOLOGICAL THEORIES

Contemporary hypotheses about neurobiological substrates of anxiety and fear focus on several interconnected subsystems of the central nervous system. One subsystem comprises noradrenergic innervation arising from cell bodies in the locus coeruleus, a bilateral nucleus of cell bodies located in the central gray matter of the isthmus on the floor of the fourth ventricle. Axons from these cells provide the main noradrenergic input to the ipsilateral cortex, cingulate gyrus, hippocampus, and cerebellum. They also impinge on cells in the hypothalamus, thalamus, septal nuclei, and other subcortical structures, where their influence is augmented by input from noradrenergic cells in the lateral tegmental nuclei. Anatomical and pharmacological manipulation of this system in animal models provide convincing evidence of its role in regulating aspects of cerebral arousal. This arousal is postulated to be experienced as vigilance, anxiety, fear, or panic, in order of increasing intensity. Hypothesized pathogenic influences on this system include genetic mechanisms, early experiences, and the interaction of the two. Workers in this area theorize that early experiences lead to structural and functional alterations in the responsivity of this system, which ultimately leads to pathological states of anxiety (3).

Another major area of investigation focuses on benzodiazepine receptors localized to central neurons. These receptors appear to be linked to a "supramolecular receptor complex" that includes a receptor for γ-aminobutyric acid (GABA) and a chloride ion channel. Binding of a benzodiazepine molecule to this receptor facilitates the ability of the GABA-receptor complex to open chloride channels, allowing negatively charged chloride ions to enter the cell and produce hyperpolarization, thereby reducing the cell's reactivity to stimulation and its likelihood of conducting an impulse. Recent autoradiographic studies have demonstrated benzodiazepine receptors in brain stem structures including the superior colliculus, the ventral nucleus of the lateral lemniscus, and the substantia nigra, all of which, together with the amygdala, comprise a component of the system that mediates the startle response. This response has been extensively studied in animal models, and pathological influences on its function have been postulated to underlie anxiety disorders in humans (4). Despite these promising beginnings, there is no accepted neurobiological theory of anxiety or anxiety disorders in humans of any age, and relatively little work in the area of aging.

DIAGNOSIS

DSM-III-R diagnostic criteria for phobic disorder, obsessive-compulsive disorder, and panic disorder are displayed in Tables 6-2, 6-3, and 6-4.

LABORATORY EVALUATION

Laboratory evaluation of the elderly patient with anxiety is aimed at ruling out physical, chemical, and iatrogenic factors that can cause or exacerbate anxiety and related symptoms. When medical evaluation reveals anxiety or its related symptoms to be caused by such factors, the correct diagnosis is organic anxiety disorder. Functional anxiety may also coexist with organic factors that exacerbate but do not cause it, in which case the correct diagnosis is anxiety disorder. Table 6-5 lists common physical conditions, chemicals, and medications that can cause anxiety. Laboratory tests should be chosen to rule out these factors.

TABLE 6-5. **Organic causes of anxiety**

Endogenous illnesses
- Hyperadrenocorticalism
- Hyperthyroidism
- Hypoadrenocorticalism
- Hypoglycemia (any cause)
- Insulinoma with hypoglycemia
- Pheochromocytoma

Medications
- Anticholinergics (atropine, scopolamine)
- Antidepressants
    Fluoxetine
    Tranylcypromine
- Caffeine
- Psychostimulants
    Amphetamine
    Cocaine
    Methylphenidate
- Sympathomimetics
    Decongestants
    Phenylephrine
    Phenylpropanolamine
    Pseudoephedrine
    Bronchodilators
    Albuterol
    Epinephrine
    Isoproterenol
    Metaproterenol
- Xanthine derivatives
    Theophylline
    Aminophylline

Medication withdrawal
- Alcohol
- Benzodiazepines, especially short-acting agents
- Other central nervous system depressants

DIFFERENTIAL DIAGNOSIS

Organic Anxiety Disorder

This condition can mimic in every way the features of functional anxiety disorder, and the diagnosis rests on identification from the history, physical examination, or laboratory tests of a specific organic factor (or factors) that is judged to be etiologically related to the disturbance. Table 6-5 lists the most common organic etiologies of anxiety. The diagnosis of organic anxiety disorder is not made during the course of delirium. Treatment of organic anxiety disorder is discussed in Chapter 7.

Mood Disorder

Anxiety is often a prominent part of major depression, dysthymia, bipolar mood disorder, and cyclothymia, and the correct diagnostic differentiation from these conditions rests on identification of the prominent and persistent alterations of mood characteristic of each of these conditions. Dysphoria, depression, and an agitated hypomanic-like state can accompany anxiety disorders, but these are generally intermittent, episodic, and self-limiting states. Because many older patients are not accustomed to introspection and may not be familiar with the appropriate psychological terms, it can be difficult to distinguish the "secondary" frustration and dysphoria associated with persistent anxiety from that characteristic of mood disorder. It is also possible, and is probably not a rare occurrence, for anxiety disorder to evolve over time into a major mood disorder.

Schizophrenia

Although the characteristic hallucinations, delusions, thought disorder, and catatonic behavior of schizophrenia and delusional disorder are clearly not a part of uncomplicated anxiety disorder, elderly patients with these conditions may be quite secretive about their psychotic experiences and can appear to be suffering from anxiety alone. Extra effort to establish rapport and develop the patient's trust can be very important in this situation; hospitalized elderly patients often connect with a particular staff member (usually on the night shift) whom they trust and with whom they will share their inner psychic content. If doubt persists, projective psychological tests (e.g., the thematic apperception test, the Rorschach test; see Chapter 3) can be of value in identifying suppressed psychotic thought content. Another potentially difficult diagnostic situation relates to the differentiation between obsessive thoughts (in obsessive-compulsive disorder) and schizophrenic delusions. DSM-III-R suggests that even when obsessions become ego-syntonic "overvalued ideas," they remain somewhat amenable to challenge by evidence or logic, allowing the clinician to distinguish them from manifestations of psychosis.

TREATMENT

PSYCHOSOCIAL-BEHAVIOR TREATMENT

Although definitive studies in geriatric patients are lacking, there is little clinical basis to doubt the efficacy of traditional psychotherapeutic approaches to anxiety in the elderly. However, cost considerations often favor use of more focused, time-limited techniques such as behavior therapies. This category includes relaxation techniques aimed at generalized reduction of muscle tension and anxiety, desensitization techniques that typically pair a state of induced relaxation with a real or imagined feared situation or object, and graded exposure approaches that attempt to gradually extinguish anxiety, fear responses, or compulsive rituals by increasingly prolonged and intense exposure to feared situations. Although studies with elderly subjects are few, clinical experience suggests that these behavior techniques can be effective with older patients, although the pace of programming may need to be adjusted, and instructions repeated or simplified. In general, the best results are obtained in patients who are capable of clearly describing the situations that provoke anxiety or ritualistic behavior. For patients whose anxiety is generalized or pervasive, techniques such as hypnosis, meditation, and guided imagery may have a role.

Most physicians who use behavior techniques in the treatment of anxiety advocate the adjunctive use of antianxiety agents along with behavior treatment; similarly, when phobic or obsessive-compulsive behaviors emerge as part of a depressive syndrome, pharmacologic treatment of depression should be initiated before or during the application of behavior therapy.

PSYCHOPHARMACOLOGIC TREATMENT

Benzodiazepines remain the treatment of choice for anxiety of acute or subacute duration (see Table 6-6). For very short-term anxiety associated with specific situations such as airplane travel, the longer-acting agents such as diazepam can be used safely; where treatment is required on a daily or near-daily basis, such as in adjustment disorder with anxiety, or in chronic generalized anxiety disorder, daily use of the longer-acting agents in elderly patients will lead to accumulation of clinically significant blood levels of long-acting active metabolites, the half-lives of most of which are several days or more. Therefore, in these situations, the shorter-acting benzodiazepines such as lorazepam or oxazepam, which undergo single-step conjugation in the liver and have no active metabolites, are preferable. These agents have the additional advantage of being relatively well tolerated by patients with even fairly advanced liver disease.

For treatment beyond 4–6 weeks, benzodiazepines may lose effectiveness, and more reliable results may be obtained with heterocyclic antidepressants such as trazodone, nortriptyline, or desipramine. Dosages are generally less than those required for treatment of depression, and peak effects on anxiety tend to occur sooner than peak antidepressant effects; otherwise, prescription follows the guidelines for treatment of mood disorder outlined in Chapter 4.

Buspirone hydrochloride, an agent recently marketed for the treatment of anxiety, has several properties that would make it an ideal agent for elderly patients. It has no sedative effects, interacts with few other medications (including alcohol), is not associated with dependence or withdrawal symptoms, and has little abuse potential. A potential disadvantage is that it has little or no acute efficacy, and usually several weeks of daily dosage are required before effects are observed. More clinical research and clinical experience with this agent will be required to precisely define its role in the treatment of anxiety in the elderly patient.

In general, neuroleptics have a very minimal role in the treatment of uncomplicated anxiety, although occasional treatment-resistant patients will respond favorably to small doses (e.g., 10–15 mg two or three times a day) of low-potency agents such as thioridazine.

TABLE 6-6. **Pharmacologic properties of benzodiazepines**

Drug	Trade name	Rate of absorption	Rate of metabolism	Elimination half-life (hours)	Therapeutic dosage range (mg/day)[a]
Chlordiazepoxide	Librium	Intermediate	Long	5–30	10–40
Diazepam	Valium	Fast	Long	20–50	2–20
Clorazepate	Tranxene	Fast	Long	36–200	7.5–30
Prazepam	Centrax	Fast	Long	36–200	20–60
Halazepam	Paxipam	Intermediate	Long	50–100	20–100
Alprazolam	Xanax	Intermediate	Intermediate	12–15	0.25–4
Lorazepam	Ativan	Intermediate	Short	10–14	0.5–6
Oxazepam	Serax	Slow	Short	5–10	15–60

[a]Approximate range; some patients may require higher or lower dosages.
Source. Adapted with permission from American Psychiatric Association: Treatments of Psychiatric Disorders: A Task Force Report of the American Psychiatric Association. Washington, DC, American Psychiatric Association, 1989, p 2040. Copyright 1989 The American Psychiatric Association.

Treatment of panic disorder is somewhat more specific. Although efficacy of alprazolam has been recently claimed, in general, benzodiazepines are relatively ineffective in abolishing panic attacks. For this purpose, tricyclic antidepressants or monoamine oxidase inhibitors are both effective; dosages are titrated to adequate symptom relief, following cautions listed in Chapter 4 for treatment of depression.

■ LATE-ONSET PSYCHOSIS

EPIDEMIOLOGY

The prevalence of late-onset psychosis is difficult to estimate because of a lack of diagnostic consistency across investigations. DSM-III-R, which may help to improve the situation, describes several psychoses that can have late-onset: schizophrenia, delusional disorder, mood disorder with psychotic features, organic hallucinosis, and organic delusional disorder. In addition, primary degenerative dementia, senile onset, and multi-infarct dementia can also be coded as "with delusions." In the National Institute of Mental Health Epidemiologic Catchment Area Program (1), 0.1% of individuals age 65 or older were diagnosed as schizophrenic with DSM-III (5) criteria, which did not allow onset of schizophrenia after the age of 45. Prevalence of psychosis associated with cognitive impairment or mood disorder was not reported. More useful estimates were provided by Leuchter and Spar (6), who reported that first onset of psychosis after age 65 was diagnosed in 8% of 880 patients admitted to a university hospital–based gerontopsychiatric unit. The diagnostic breakdown was as follows: 3.4% had organic mental disorder (mainly primary degenerative or multi-infarct dementia) with psychosis, 2.8% had mood disorder with psychosis, and 1.7% had disorders that would be diagnosed by DSM-III-R criteria as schizophrenia (10 of 15 patients) or delusional disorder (4 of 15 patients). A similar study by Craig and Bregman (7) found that 2.1% of 658 hospitalized elderly patients with a (DSM-III) diagnosis of schizophrenia or paranoid disorder had onset of symptoms after age 65.

CLINICAL PRESENTATION

The clinical presentation of late-onset psychosis depends in large part on the underlying diagnosis. Mood disorder with psychosis is described in Chapter 3 and dementia with psychosis in Chapter 5; the remainder of this chapter will focus on late-onset schizophrenia and delusional disorder.

PATHOGENESIS

PSYCHODYNAMIC THEORIES

A number of plausible psychodynamic hypotheses have been proposed to explain the development of delusions in mental illness, although none has focused on late-onset disorders. These hypotheses assume that delusions are "secondary," functioning to help maintain psychic equilibrium threatened by peculiar or frightening experiences. Applying this principle, the common delusion expressed by demented patients that people are stealing things from them becomes an "explanation" for the disappearance and reappearance of items that are actually misplaced. The delusion allows the individual to be able to avoid the awareness of declining memory function. Similarly, delusions of bodily malfunction ("I can't eat because the food doesn't go into my stomach anymore") and delusional guilt ("The President has lost his veto power and the Communists are going to take over because of me") commonly seen in psychotic major depression help the individual to explain and understand his or her pervasive sense of dysphoria, degradation, and helplessness. In late-onset schizophrenia and delusional disorder, wherein intellectual deficits and mood disturbance are absent, the primary stimulus for the development of delusions has been postulated to be an inner sense of meaninglessness or insignificance, or a feeling that the environment has changed in some subtle and threatening way. Delusions tend to be of a paranoid nature in both instances; in the former, delusions embody a sense of grandiose status: "The actions of many other people are oriented around me, so I must be a powerful and important person." In the latter, the "changed" environment is explained by the covert, usually hostile actions of others. Delusional beliefs often seem designed to explain hallucinatory experiences; for example, "The neighbors are pumping poison gas into my apartment" is a belief that might accompany olfactory hallucinations. Psychodynamic explanations of hallucinations, catatonic behavior, and flat affect, each of which is a DSM-III-R criterion for schizophrenia, are less completely articulated in the literature.

NEUROBIOLOGICAL THEORIES

Neurobiological explanations of delusions and hallucinations depend on the specific organic etiology. An analogy has been drawn between the dopaminergic hyperactivity postulated to underlie functional psychosis and the organic psychosis associated with chronic ingestion of dopaminergic agents such as amphetamine or cocaine. Similarly, the psychotic symptoms associated with ingestion of serotonergic hallucinogens like LSD have been proposed as a partial "model" of functional psychosis; however, no widely accepted theory relating naturally occurring to drug-induced psychosis has been articulated. Neurobiological explanations of psychosis associated with structural lesions of the brain are even less well developed, but should benefit from contemporary attention to the preliminary task of correlating mental manifestations with brain pathology (8).

DIAGNOSIS

DSM-III-R diagnostic criteria for schizophrenia and delusional disorder are displayed in Tables 6-7 and 6-8.

DIFFERENTIAL DIAGNOSIS

As indicated above, the major diagnostic entities to be ruled out before making the diagnosis of late-onset schizophrenia or delusional disorder are mood disorder with psychosis and dementia with psychosis. Delirium, particularly if induced by medications, should also be considered.

In psychotic mood disorder, sadness, dysphoria, anhedonia, and irritability are usually apparent enough to lead diagnostic efforts in the right direction; when these features are obscured by psychotic manifestations, the diagnosis may rest on identification of the characteristic neurovegetative signs and symptoms of de-

TABLE 6-7. **Diagnostic criteria for schizophrenia**

A. Presence of characteristic psychotic symptoms in the active phase: either (1), (2), or (3) for at least 1 week (unless the symptoms are successfully treated):
   (1) Two of the following:
      (a) Delusions
      (b) Prominent hallucinations
      (c) Incoherence or marked loosening of associations
      (d) Catatonic behavior
      (e) Flat or grossly inappropriate affect
   (2) Bizarre delusions
   (3) Prominent hallucinations of a voice with content having no apparent relation to depression or elation, or a voice keeping up a running commentary on the person's behavior or thoughts, or two or more voices conversing with each other

B. During the course of the disturbance, functioning in work, social relations, and self-care is markedly impaired.

C. Schizoaffective and mood disorder with psychotic features have been ruled out.

D. Continuous signs of the disturbance for at least 6 months.

E. It cannot be established that an organic factor initiated and maintained the disturbance.

Source. Adapted with permission from American Psychiatric Association: Diagnostic and Statistical Manual of Mental Disorders, 3rd Edition, Revised. Washington, DC, American Psychiatric Association, 1987, pp 194–195. Copyright 1987 The American Psychiatric Association.

pression and careful determination of a sequence of onset of symptoms in which mood and neurovegetative changes occur before delusions and hallucinations. Late-onset hypomania and mania can present a picture very similar to that of schizophrenia and delusional disorder (9). Again, correct diagnosis may require a detailed history obtained from multiple sources, including old medical records, as well as inpatient observation. Dementia with psychosis may be identified by mental status examination supplemented with neuropsychological tests (see Chapter 5). It is important to remember that test performance in the absence of organic brain disease may be impaired if attention, concentration, and motivation are negatively impacted by functional illness. Accord-

TABLE 6-8. **Diagnostic criteria for delusional disorder**

A. Nonbizarre delusion(s) of at least 1 month's duration.

B. Auditory or visual hallucinations, if present, are not prominent.

C. Apart from the delusion(s) or its ramifications, behavior is not obviously odd or bizarre.

D. If a major depressive or manic syndrome has been present during the delusional disturbance, the total duration of all episodes of the mood syndrome has been brief relative to the total duration of the delusional disturbance.

E. Has never met criterion A for schizophrenia, and it cannot be established that an organic factor initiated and maintained the disturbance.

Source. Adapted with permission from American Psychiatric Association: Diagnostic and Statistical Manual of Mental Disorders, 3rd Edition, Revised. Washington, DC, American Psychiatric Association, 1987, p 202. Copyright 1987 The American Psychiatric Association.

ingly, retesting after these symptoms are at least partly controlled may avoid false-positive findings of organicity.

Finally, delirium is rarely mistaken for schizophrenia or delusional disorder, but medications or combinations of medications that produce psychomotor slowing and toxic hallucinations (a good example is low-potency neuroleptic medications with potent central anticholinergic effects) can lead to this potentially hazardous misdiagnosis.

TREATMENT

PSYCHOSOCIAL THERAPY

Because of the unpredictability of the behavior of acutely psychotic elderly patients, it is generally advisable to treat them in the hospital. In this setting, individual supportive psychotherapy aimed at building trust, facilitating the flow of clinical data from the patient, and maximizing compliance with somatic therapy can be an effective component of the overall treatment program. An effective therapeutic stance to take toward the patient's delusional belief is "respectful disagreement," wherein the therapist does not claim to share the patient's false belief, but avoids confrontation or argument with its content. Psychotic patients generally realize that others do not agree with their beliefs, and they may become suspicious and distrustful of the treating professional who does. On the other hand, open disagreement invites the patient to incorporate the therapist into the delusion, thereby thwarting efforts to establish a mutually respectful, trusting relationship.

Although some elderly patients are capable of some detachment from their delusions and can gain insight into their defensive function, insight-oriented psychotherapeutic approaches are usually discouraged in favor of approaches that focus on more dynamically superficial content, such as conscious concerns and feelings. In this regard, psychotic patients often refuse to cooperate with treatment aimed at the delusions or hallucinations per se, in which case an effective approach is to emphasize the accompanying anxiety, fear, sleeplessness, or anhedonia.

Group therapy is generally of little value in the acute phase of psychotic illness, although some patients are able to use the group situation to initiate social contact with other patients and appear to benefit indirectly.

Family therapy may be extremely useful, particularly in situations wherein family members have been alienated by psychotic behavior. Although sessions without the patient can be productive, it is advisable to invite the patient's participation each time. Work with family members focuses on education about the patient's condition, its natural history and prognosis, and details of the treatment plan; the family therapist also attempts to enlist family support for the inpatient and outpatient components of the treatment plan.

PSYCHOPHARMACOTHERAPY

The mainstays of treatment for late-onset schizophrenia and delusional disorder are high-potency neuroleptic medications, of which haloperidol, fluphenazine, and thiothixene are representative agents. Dosages required to achieve symptom remission vary considerably, but a starting dose of 1 mg twice daily of haloperidol or fluphenazine, twice that for thiothixene, is appropriate for most elderly individuals. If significant side effects do not occur, these dosages are supplemented by similar doses prescribed "as needed" every 2–4 hours for agitation, hallucinations, or delusion-driven behavior (e.g., the patient won't eat because the food "comes from the toilet" or is "poisoned"). In this manner, the standing daily dosage is gradually increased by an amount equal to the average daily "prn" dosage until behavior disruption, hallucinations, and delusion-driven behavior are under control. Because delusional content may persist for weeks or months after delusions are emotionally and behaviorally "empty," it is not practical to use delusional content as a target symptom of acute therapy. After acute symptomatology subsides, gradual dosage reduction can be undertaken until symptom breakthrough occurs, at which point the dosage is increased slightly and maintained. Medium- and low-potency agents are equally effective in equipotent dosages, but cause side effects that are much less well tolerated by elderly individuals than the mild extrapyramidal effects associated with the higher potency agents. Table 6-9 displays dose equivalences and relative side-effect potencies of the commonly prescribed neuroleptics.

Benzodiazepine hypnotics and anxiolytics, particularly those with short half-lives, may be used adjunctly as needed, as may cyclic antidepressants when significant mood disorder is present. Side effects associated with this approach are usually minimal. Mild extrapyramidal symptoms of akinesia and cogwheel rigidity may be observed but are usually not associated with subjective distress in elderly patients. On the other hand, akathisia and daytime drowsiness, sometimes occurring simultaneously, can be a problem and may require dosage reduction. Adjunctive treatment with lorazepam or other short-acting benzodiazepines often allows the total dosage of neuroleptic to be reduced below levels that cause these side effects. One or two doses of antiparkinsonian agents such as benztropine and trihexyphenidyl hydrochloride may be useful for diagnostic purposes when akathisia is suspected, but chronic administration of these agents should be avoided whenever possible because of the susceptibility of elderly patients to memory impairment, confusion, and anticholinergic delirium.

Alternatively, clonazepam, which produces no extrapyramidal side effects, may be effective in controlling agitation and hallucinations, but seems to be less effective than neuroleptic medications in reversing thought disorder and delusions. A typi-

158

TABLE 6–9. **Antipsychotic drugs, dose equivalences, and side-effect profile**

Drug	Equivalent dose	Sedation	Anticholinergic effects	Extrapyramidal effect[a]	Hypotensive effects
Chlorpromazine [b]	100	++	++	++	+++ (im)
Thioridazine [c]	100	+++	+++	+	++
Loxapine	15	+	+	++	+
Molindone	10	++	0	+	0
Perphenazine	8	++	+/0	+++	+
Trifluoperazine	5	+	+	++	+
Thiothixene	5	+	+/0	++	++
Haloperidol	2	+	0	+++	+/0
Fluphenazine	2	+	+/0	+++	+

[a] Includes acute dystonias, pseudoparkinsonism, akathisia, and perioral tremor ("rabbit syndrome").
[b] Five percent of patients develop urticaria or dermatitis.
[c] Maximal dose is 800 mg/day; higher doses may cause pigmentary retinopathy.
Source. Adapted from Wise MG, Rundell JR: Concise Guide to Consultation Psychiatry. Washington, DC, American Psychiatric Press, 1988, p 30. Copyright 1988 American Psychiatric Press.

cal starting dosage of clonazepam is 0.5 mg administered orally three times per day, which can be increased up to threefold. At these dosages, side effects are usually limited to sedation, but the risk of blood dyscrasia necessitates a pretreatment complete blood count and periodic retesting.

■ REFERENCES

1. Regier DA, Boyd JH, Burke JD Jr, et al: One month prevalence of mental disorders in the United States. Arch Gen Psychiatry 45:977–986, 1988
2. American Psychiatric Association: Diagnostic and Statistical Manual of Mental Disorders, 3rd Edition, Revised. Washington, DC, American Psychiatric Association, 1987
3. Redmond DE Jr: Studies of the nucleus locus coeruleus in monkeys and hypotheses for neuropsychopharmacology, in Psychopharmacology: The Third Generation of Progress. Edited by Meltzer HY. New York, Raven, 1987, pp 967–975
4. Hommer DW, Skolnick P, Paul DM: The benzodiazepine/GABA receptor complex and anxiety, in Psychopharmacology: The Third Generation of Progress. Edited by Meltzer HY. New York, Raven, 1987, pp 977–983
5. American Psychiatric Association: Diagnostic and Statistical Manual of Mental Disorders, 3rd Edition. Washington, DC, American Psychiatric Association, 1980
6. Leuchter A, Spar JE: The late-onset psychoses: clinical and diagnostic features. J Nerv Ment Dis 173:488–493, 1985
7. Craig TJ, Bregman Z: Late onset schizophrenia-like illness. J Am Geriatr Soc 36:104–107, 1988
8. Cummings JL: Organic delusions: phenomenology, anatomical correlations, and review. Br J Psychiatry 146:184–197, 1985
9. Spar JE, Ford CV, Liston E: Bipolar affective disorder in aged patients. J Clin Psychiatry 40:504–507, 1979

■ ADDITIONAL READING

Busse EW, Blazer DG (eds): Geriatric Psychiatry. Washington, DC, American Psychiatric Press, 1989

7 OTHER COMMON MENTAL DISORDERS OF THE ELDERLY

■ SLEEP DISORDERS

INSOMNIA

Complaints of inadequate amount or quality of sleep are extremely common in elderly patients and pose a particular diagnostic challenge. The differential diagnosis of insomnia in the elderly includes

- *Normal aging changes in sleep.* In general, with advancing age, sleep becomes more fragmented; more time is required to fall asleep, and there are more awakenings, relatively less deep (stage 4) sleep, and a tendency to spend more time in bed. Figure 7-1 displays the changes in sleep architecture in elderly patients compared with adults and children. The subjective impression produced by these changes is unsatisfying sleep, which may be reported as insomnia; it is not uncommon for elderly hospitalized patients to report not sleeping at all despite nursing observations of 6–8 hours of apparent sleep, complete with snoring.
- *Insomnia associated with mental illness.* Almost all of the major syndromes discussed in this book are associated with sleep disturbance, including anxiety disorders, mood disorders, dementia and delirium, psychosis, and adjustment disorder. To this list must be added the normal disruptions in mental life occasioned by stressful or grief-producing situations.
- *Insomnia associated with physical illness.* Physical conditions associated with pain, such as arthritis, or with difficulty breathing, such as congestive heart failure or chronic obstructive pulmonary disease, can severely disturb sleep; frequent awakenings may also be associated with urinary obstruction secondary to prostatism or chronic urinary tract infection. Nocturnal myoclonus and sleep apnea are relatively uncommon physical conditions that present as insomnia. Sleep apnea has been found in about 30–40% of elderly patients evaluated in sleep

laboratories and is typically associated with obesity and snoring. Nocturnal myoclonus, usually manifested as leg twitches and jerks, is diagnosed somewhat less frequently and may be observed without the benefit of sophisticated electronic equip-

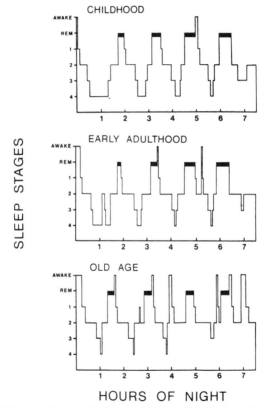

FIGURE 7-1. **Changes in sleep architecture in elderly patients compared with adults and children.** Reprinted with permission from Hauri P: The Sleep Disorders, 2nd Edition. Kalamazoo, MI, The Upjohn Company, 1982.

ment. Muscle movements that cause brief awakenings are most likely to be diagnostic of this condition.

- *Insomnia associated with medications.* Sympathomimetic agents (including decongestants and bronchodilators), methylxanthine derivatives such as theophylline and aminophylline, psychostimulants, certain antidepressants (fluoxetine, sometimes protriptyline and tranylcypromine), and medications containing caffeine (as well as caffeine-containing beverages like coffee and many cola drinks) can interfere with sleep, particularly if ingested late in the evening. There is also experimental and clinical evidence that most, if not all, hypnotic medications can produce sleep disturbance after prolonged use (sometimes in as little as 3 weeks of nightly ingestion) or during the acute withdrawal phase after repeated ingestion (the so-called rebound effect).

- *Primary insomnia.* When the above causes of insomnia have been ruled out, the proper diagnosis is primary insomnia, the DSM-III-R (1) diagnostic criteria for which are given in Table 7-1.

TABLE 7-1. **Diagnostic criteria for insomnia**

Diagnostic Criteria for Insomnia Disorders

A. Difficulty in initiating or maintaining sleep, or nonrestorative sleep

B. The disturbance in A occurs at least three times a week for at least 1 month and results in either a complaint of daytime fatigue or the observation by others of some symptom that is attributable to the sleep disturbance, e.g., irritability or impaired daytime functioning.

C. Occurrence not exclusively during the course of sleep-wake schedule disorder or a parasomnia.

Diagnostic Criteria for Primary Insomnia

Insomnia disorder, as defined by criteria A, B, and C above, that apparently is not maintained by any other mental disorder or any known organic factor such as a physical disorder, a psychoactive substance use disorder, or a medication.

Source. Adapted with permission from American Psychiatric Association: Diagnostic and Statistical Manual of Mental Disorders, 3rd Edition, Revised. Washington, DC, American Psychiatric Association, 1987, pp 299–300, 301. Copyright 1987 The American Psychiatric Association.

TREATMENT

General Considerations

In light of the above differential diagnosis of insomnia, it is important whenever possible to treat mental and physical illness and to adjust the type, dosage, and timing of medications that can cause insomnia, before prescribing hypnotic agents. Of the physical illnesses that can disturb sleep, it is particularly important to identify and treat sleep apnea, as prescription of sedative-hypnotic agents can exacerbate this condition and create a potentially lethal situation. Similarly, optimization of "sleep hygiene" should always be attempted before hypnotic agents are prescribed for other than occasional use (2). Table 7-2 lists the most important factors to consider.

Psychopharmacologic Treatment

Benzodiazepine anxiolytic and hypnotic medications (see Table 7-3) are the agents of choice for elderly patients with primary insomnia. Although Table 7-3 lists only three benzodiazepines that are specifically marketed for inducing sleep, all agents of this class have hypnotic activity and are essentially interchangeable, even though minor interindividual differences in susceptibility to one or more of their effects are the rule. For occasional use, almost any of the available agents are effective, but most elderly patients will experience less morning "hangover" with the short-acting agents such as temazepam, lorazepam, or oxazepam than with the long-acting agents such as diazepam or flurazepam. In this regard, alprazolam is intermediate in duration of action and in desirability, whereas triazolam is very short acting but is to be avoided because of its propensity to cause ataxia, paradoxical agitation, and mild but sometimes disturbing amnesia in some elderly patients. Nonbenzodiazepine agents have few advantages and should generally also be avoided, but are listed in Table 7-3 for completeness. In particular, the popular practice of prescribing antihistamines such as diphenhydramine is not recommended because of the central anticholinergic potency of medications in this category. Some elderly patients will experience improved sleep with the amino acid L-tryptophan, which can be administered in dosages of 1–5 g. However, this amount may cost several

TABLE 7-2. **Eleven rules for better sleep hygiene**

1. Sleep as much as needed to feel refreshed and healthy during the following day, but not more. Curtailing the time in bed seems to solidify sleep; excessively long times in bed seem related to fragmented and shallow sleep.

2. A regular arousal time in the morning strengthens circadian cycling and leads to regular times of sleep onset.

3. A steady daily amount of exercise probably deepens sleep; occasional exercise does not necessarily improve sleep the following night.

4. Occasional loud noises (e.g., aircraft flyovers) disturb sleep even in people who are not awakened by noises and cannot remember them in the morning. Sound-attenuated bedrooms may help those who must sleep close to noise.

5. Although excessively warm rooms disturb sleep, there is no evidence that an excessively cold room solidifies sleep.

6. Hunger may disturb sleep; a light snack may help sleep.

7. An occasional sleeping pill may be of some benefit, but chronic use of medications is ineffective in most insomniacs.

8. Caffeine in the evening disturbs sleep, even in those who feel it does not.

9. Alcohol helps tense people fall asleep easily, but the ensuing sleep is then fragmented.

10. People who feel angry and frustrated because they cannot sleep should not try harder and harder to fall asleep but should turn on the light and do something different.

11. The chronic use of tobacco disturbs sleep.

Source. Reprinted with permission from Hauri P: The Sleep Disorders, 2nd Edition. Kalamazoo, MI, The Upjohn Company, 1982.

dollars per dose and is usually not as effective as the other agents listed. Recent concern about a possible association with eosinophilia myalgia syndrome also militates against the use of L-tryptophan.

For chronic use, the short-acting agents named above are greatly preferable to long-acting agents because of the risk, with

TABLE 7-3. **Sedative-hypnotics with dosage and duration of action**

Generic name (trade name)	Dosage	Duration of action
Benzodiazepine hypnotics		
Flurazepam (Dalmane)	15–30 mg	Long
Temazepam (Restoril)	15–30 mg	Short
Triazolam (Halcion)	0.125–0.250 mg	Ultrashort
Benzodiazepine anxiolytics		
Lorazepam (Ativan)	0.5–2 mg	Short
Oxazepam (Serax)	15–30 mg	Short
Diazepam (Valium)	2.5–5 mg	Long
Alprazolam (Xanax)	5–1.0 mg	Short
Barbiturates		
Pentobarbital (Nembutal)	50–100 mg	Intermediate
Secobarbital (Seconal)	50–500 mg	Intermediate
Others		
Chloral hydrate (many)	500–1,000 mg	Intermediate
Glutethimide (Doriden)	125–250 mg	Intermediate
Methyprylon (Noludar)	100–200 mg	Intermediate
L-Tryptophan	1–5 g	Intermediate

the latter, of building up potentially intoxicating blood levels of very long-acting active metabolites. The following case is illustrative:

A 76-year-old woman was admitted to the hospital for evaluation of mental cloudiness and lethargy. Comprehensive medical and neurological workup failed to reveal a cause of her symptoms, and the fact that she had started taking 5 mg of diazepam per night for sleep about 2 months before admission was initially ignored. Subsequent consultation with a geriatric psychopharmacologist led to discontinuation of the diazepam and rapid amelioration of her symptoms.

Because most hypnotic agents begin to lose effectiveness after several weeks of nightly ingestion, it is important to provide detailed instructions on their use, with emphasis on the advantages of irregular administration. Some clinicians attempt to avoid the development of tolerance by prescribing two or three different benzodiazepine agents at the same time, with instructions to the patient to switch back and forth between the medications on a weekly basis. Although this approach has been successful in selected instances, no formal research data supporting this practice have yet been published.

■ SUBSTANCE ABUSE

ALCOHOLISM

EPIDEMIOLOGY

Estimates of the prevalence of alcohol abuse in community-dwelling elderly range from 3 to 3.7% of men over age 65, as reported in a 1984 survey (3), to those reported in the recent National Institute of Mental Health Epidemiologic Catchment Area survey (4), which found that only 0.9% of men (and no women) over the age of 65 (compared to 2.8% for men and women of all ages combined), met DSM-III (5) diagnostic criteria for alcohol abuse/dependence. Although data from different surveys disagree on absolute numbers, probably based in part on differences in diagnostic criteria, it appears that the rate of problem drinking significantly declines sometime after mid-life (i.e., the 50s) into and through the 70s. Several factors have been proposed to account for this phenomenon: attrition of alcohol abusers by early, alcohol-related death; underreporting of alcohol-related symptoms (which are obscured by symptoms of other age-related illnesses or the effects of aging itself); and underestimating community prevalence of alcoholism because many elderly alcoholic patients are institutionalized for other reasons and are therefore missed by community surveys, or because diagnoses are based on criteria that assume that the individual being diagnosed has a "normal" work and social life, which may not hold for many elderly individuals living in the community. A somewhat more morbid possibility, and one for which there is some evidence (discussed below), is that older individuals, typically seen as unlikely candidates for drug abuse, find it easier to obtain sedative-hypnotic medications from doctors and are able to replace some alcohol with these agents and thereby partially trade one addiction for another. Finally, it is possible that people in fact "get over" alcoholism through some natural process leading to spontaneous recovery. Whichever is the true explanation, it must be a common occurrence, as there is evidence that over one-third of elderly alcoholic patients begin their pathological substance use after age 60 (6); accordingly, prevalence data reported above must overestimate the number of alcoholic patients who have persisted in pathological drinking from middle age.

DIAGNOSTIC CRITERIA

DSM-III-R distinguishes alcohol dependence, which is defined in Table 7-4, from the less severe syndrome of alcohol abuse, which

TABLE 7-4. Diagnostic criteria for psychoactive substance dependence

A. At least three of the following:

(1) Substance often taken in larger amounts or over a longer period than the person intended

(2) Persistent desire or one or more unsuccessful efforts to cut down or control substance use

(3) A great deal of time spent in activities necessary to get the substance, taking the substance, or recovering from its effects

(4) Frequent intoxication or withdrawal symptoms when expected to fulfill major role obligations at work, school, or home

(5) Important social, occupational, or recreational activities given up or reduced because of substance use

(6) Continued substance use despite knowledge of having a social, psychological, or physical problem that is caused or exacerbated by the use of the substance

(7) Marked tolerance: need for at least a 50% increase in amount ingested in order to achieve intoxication or desired effect, or markedly diminished effect with continued use of the same amount

(8) Characteristic withdrawal symptoms

(9) Substance often taken to relieve or avoid withdrawal symptoms

Source. Adapted with permission from American Psychiatric Association: Diagnostic and Statistical Manual of Mental Disorders, 3rd Edition, Revised. Washington, DC, American Psychiatric Association, 1987, pp 167–168. Copyright 1987 The American Psychiatric Association.

is defined in Table 7-5. Although these criteria are intended to apply throughout the life span, the inapplicability of some of them to elderly persons should be kept in mind.

ASSOCIATED PSYCHIATRIC CONDITIONS

Because acute consumption of alcohol is known to impair cognitive function, and chronic consumption has been associated with a reversible dementia, it is not surprising that authors of one recent study found that almost one-half of a group of 216 elderly patients hospitalized for alcoholism had some form of organic brain syndrome (7). Similarly, the known central nervous system depressant effects of alcohol undoubtedly contributed to the 12% prevalence of mood disorder in the same sample. Although the precise relationship between alcohol consumption and disorders of mood and cognition remains to be determined, it is important to screen carefully for both conditions; even mild degrees of cognitive impairment could interfere with treatment, and symptoms of underlying mood disorder can easily be obscured by symptoms related to alcohol ingestion. If depression is present, antidepressant therapy can usually be delayed until several weeks

TABLE 7-5. **Diagnostic criteria for psychoactive substance abuse**

A. A maladaptive pattern of psychoactive substance use indicated by at least one of the following:
  (1) Continued use despite knowledge of having a persistent or recurrent social, occupational, psychological, or physical problem that is caused or exacerbated by use of the psychoactive substance
  (2) Recurrent use in situations in which use is physically hazardous

B. Some symptoms of the disturbance have persisted for at least 1 month, or have occurred repeatedly over a longer period of time.

C. Never met the criteria for psychoactive substance dependence for this substance.

Source. Adapted with permission from American Psychiatric Association: Diagnostic and Statistical Manual of Mental Disorders, 3rd Edition, Revised. Washington, DC, American Psychiatric Association, 1987, p 169. Copyright 1987 The American Psychiatric Association.

after detoxification, as there is evidence that depressive symptoms will spontaneously resolve in a significant proportion of cases.

TREATMENT

Principles of treatment are generally the same as those appropriate for middle-aged alcoholic patients; treatment programs containing elements of traditional psychotherapy, behavior therapy, and administration of disulfiram have been successful. Published data suggest that elderly alcoholic patients respond as well or better to such treatment, particularly if they are late-onset drinkers (8).

OTHER PSYCHOACTIVE SUBSTANCE ABUSE

EPIDEMIOLOGY

Although relatively little attention has been given to this phenomenon, there is increasing evidence that substance abuse is a clinically significant problem among elderly Americans. For the most part, use of "street" drugs does not appear to be a major concern; rather, the clinician must consider a broader category of drug "misuse," including overutilization and inappropriate mixing of psychoactive and nonpsychoactive prescription and over-the-counter agents, failure to use necessary medications as prescribed, and occasional abuse of illegitimate agents. The magnitude of this problem is unknown, although several recent studies suggest that it could affect as many as 14–25% of elderly outpatients seen in psychiatric settings (7,9).

COMMON PATTERNS OF ABUSE

Table 7-6 lists agents that are abused by elderly patients and that should be inquired about in any suspect cases. In addition to simple over- or underuse of prescribed and over-the-counter drugs, the clinician should inquire about timing of drug ingestions, because significant problems could arise from combining several agents in the following list:

- Benzodiazepine anxiolytics and antihistamines (additive sedation)

TABLE 7-6. **Psychoactive substances abused by elderly patients**

- Sedative-hypnotics
    Barbiturates
    Benzodiazepines
    Chloral hydrate
    Over-the-counter antihistamines

- Narcotic analgesics
    Codeine
    Oxycodone
    Propoxyphene

- Nonnarcotic analgesics
    Acetaminophen
    Aspirin
    Other nonsteroidal anti-inflammatory agents

- Cold preparations containing anticholinergic antihistamines
    Chlorpheniramine
    Diphenhydramine

- Cold preparations containing stimulating sympathomimetics
    Ephedrine
    Phenylephrine
    Phenylpropanolamine
    Pseudoephedrine

- Over-the-counter products containing caffeine or alcohol

- Narcotic analgesics and antihistamines (additive sedation, constipation)
- Decongestants and caffeine (additive stimulation)

TREATMENT

The key to treatment of elderly substance abusers is recognition by the patient and the primary physician that a problem exists. Once the problem has been identified and acknowledged, the specific approach is dictated by clinical circumstances. Detoxification in the hospital is often the first step and should be considered whenever drug effects are obvious and the precise identity of the drugs and their dosages cannot be reliably ascertained. After that step, it is worthwhile to attempt to enlist spouses, other family members, the patient's other physicians, and, where possible, the local druggist to help maintain surveillance and control of availability of substances. Sponsors of board-and-care homes and retirement hotel administrators are often willing and able to assist in this manner as well. A firm therapeutic alliance with the patient, in the context of which the patient's fears that his or her real or imagined symptoms will go untreated if abused substances are not available, can be extremely important and may in itself obviate the need for further intervention.

■ SEXUAL DYSFUNCTION

SEXUAL DYSFUNCTION AND NORMAL AGING CHANGES

In general, sexual dysfunction is diagnosed on the basis of reduced function in one or more of the first three phases of the sexual response cycle: the phase of desire (DSM-III-R hypoactive sexual desire disorder), followed by the excitement phase (DSM-III-R male erectile disorder, DSM-III-R female sexual arousal disorder), followed by orgasm (DSM-III-R inhibited [male or female] orgasm). Because normal aging is associated with reduced function in all three areas, particularly in men, diagnosis of the above sexual dysfunctions in elderly patients requires that the clinician take normal aging changes into account. However, because reliable age-adjusted norms have not been published, the clinician must determine appropriate treatment goals in each case based on the patient's past level of function as tempered by realistic expectations and awareness of limitations.

Most elderly men can continue sexual activity through their 80s, but should expect that sexual desire will gradually diminish, sexual arousal will take more time and more stimulation, erections will be softer and not last as long, ejaculation may be diminished in vigor, and orgasm may not occur every time they have sex. Because of the natural lengthening of the plateau phase of arousal, premature ejaculation is somewhat less likely to occur late in life, but can occur in men of any age. Women may notice reduced vaginal lubrication (which can contribute to the development of the sexual pain disorders dyspareunia and vaginismus) and reduced desire, whereas the ability to have orgasm is more inconsistently affected, with some reporting increased ease of orgasm with age.

SEXUAL DYSFUNCTION AND PHYSICAL ILLNESS

One of the most common causes of physiologic erectile dysfunction in men is prostate surgery, with perineal prostatectomy the most likely cause of impotence, followed by retropubic prostatectomy, followed by transurethral prostatectomy. Still, with recent technical modifications, about two-thirds of men remain potent after retropubic procedures. Diabetes, renal disease, cardiac disease, colorectal and other cancers, and stroke have also been associated with sexual dysfunction and should be taken into account in the evaluation of sexual complaints by elderly men.

SEXUAL DYSFUNCTION AND MEDICATIONS

The worst offenders vis-à-vis sexual dysfunction appear to be antihypertensive medications, particularly guanethidine, methyldopa, clonidine, and the beta-blockers, all of which can impair erectile and ejaculatory function. Cyclic antidepressants and neuroleptics have also been implicated in erectile and ejaculatory dysfunction, and cyclic antidepressants and monoamine oxidase inhibitors can also cause anorgasmia in men and women. Trazodone has been reported in a relatively small number of cases to cause painful and prolonged erection (priapism) that can require surgical reduction and result in permanent damage. Although is not clear whether age is a risk factor for these adverse drug effects, a complete sexual history should address the potential contribution of these agents, and dosage adjustment or replacement should be attempted before more specific therapy is prescribed.

■ PSYCHIATRIC SYMPTOMS RELATED TO PHYSICAL ILLNESS

ORGANIC MOOD SYNDROME

Mania secondary to medications and endogenous physical illness and depression secondary to medications are discussed in Chapter 3. The endogenous illnesses that have been associated with depression are listed in Table 7-7. Of those listed, structural lesions of the brain are probably more likely to cause depression in a patient with no prior history of mood disorder, whereas the other causes listed appear to be less "potent" and more often cause depression in patients with a past history of mood disorder (10).

Treatment of organic mood syndrome is a two-phase process. First, discontinuation of medications suspected to be causing the

TABLE 7-7. **Physical illnesses that can cause depression**

- Endocrine disorders
    Hyperadrenocorticalism
    Hyperparathyroidism
    Hyperthyroidism
    Hypoadrenocorticalism
    Hypothyroidism

- Neoplastic disorders
    Brain tumor, especially of frontal lobe
    Cancer of pancreas
    Metastatic cancer to bone, with elevated serum calcium

- Neurologic conditions
    Epilepsy
    Huntington's chorea
    Multiple sclerosis
    Stroke, especially left hemisphere

- Others
    Vitamin B_{12} or folate deficiency
    Systemic lupus erythematosus
    Viral illness

mood syndrome and appropriate therapy of endocrinologic and other endogenous illnesses listed in Table 7-7 may suffice to reverse the syndrome. When these measures are ineffective, the second phase of treatment may proceed according to the guidelines presented in Chapter 4 for functional mood disorder.

ORGANIC PERSONALITY SYNDROME

Although personality changes are extremely common in dementia and are often seen in association with several of the major syndromes discussed in this book, organic personality syndrome per se is relatively rare. DSM-III-R criteria for this syndrome are listed in Table 7-8, where it can be seen that the presence of delirium or dementia rules this condition out. Still, personality syndrome as described in DSM-III-R has been described in connection with trauma, stroke, or tumor affecting the frontal lobes of the brain. According to Benson and Blumer (11), damage to the prefrontal convexities is associated with apathetic with-

TABLE 7-8. Diagnostic criteria for organic personality syndrome

A. A persistent personality disturbance, either lifelong or representing a change or accentuation of a previously characteristic trait, involving at least one of the following:
  (1) Affective instability
  (2) Recurrent outbursts of aggression or rage grossly out of proportion to precipitating stressors
  (3) Markedly impaired social judgment
  (4) Marked apathy and indifference
  (5) Suspiciousness or paranoid ideation

B. There is evidence from the history, physical examination, or laboratory tests of a specific organic factor (or factors) judged to be etiologically related to the disturbance.

C. Not occurring exclusively during the curse of delirium, and does not meet the criteria for dementia.

drawal, psychomotor slowness, and social indifference, whereas damage to the orbital surface of the frontal lobe is more likely to be associated with anger, poor impulse control, and socially inappropriate behavior. Obviously, patients with the former syndrome are most likely to be misdiagnosed as depressed, whereas those with the latter may be seen as hypomanic. The primary author (J.E.S.) has administered electroconvulsive therapy to two patients with apathetic frontal lobe personality syndrome wherein the possibility of superimposed depressive disorder was significant enough to warrant a treatment trial. Of several hundred depressed elderly patients similarly treated, these were the only two who sustained absolutely no benefit from electroconvulsive therapy. In general, treatment of organic personality syndrome is aimed at amelioration of the specific organic factor judged to be etiologic in each case.

ORGANIC DELUSIONAL SYNDROME AND ORGANIC HALLUCINOSIS

A long list of organic factors have been identified as capable of causing hallucinations or delusions. A review by Plotkin (12) suggests that the most likely organic causes of delusions in elderly patients are cerebral lesions associated with stroke or trauma, particularly if the temporal lobe and limbic structures are affected; some specific delusions have also been observed in patients with damage to occipital lobe (denial of blindness) and parietal lobe (denial of hemiparesis). Blindness and deafness have been associated with visual and auditory hallucinations, and partial complex seizures have been associated with olfactory hallucinations and delusions. Alcoholic hallucinosis is a specific syndrome that occurs within 2–3 days after termination of drinking. In this syndrome, frightening auditory or visual, sometimes tactile, hallucinations occur in an otherwise clear sensorium and are typically accompanied by persecutory delusions.

The differential diagnosis of organic hallucinosis or organic delusional syndrome includes functional psychosis, dementia, and delirium. In most cases, a complete medical evaluation will reveal the organic factor(s) judged to be etiologically related to the disturbance, allowing functional psychosis to be ruled out. In dementia, cognitive disturbance will be present, and in delirium, there will be prominent deficits in attention and concentration, sometimes frank clouding of consciousness. Inasmuch as sensory deficits have been cited as contributing factors in the development of functional psychosis in elderly patients, the correct diagnosis of a psychotic patient with sensory loss may be difficult to determine with confidence.

Treatment of organic psychosis is much the same as treatment of organic mood disorder; that is, potential exogenous causes are removed, potential endogenous causes are appropriately treated, and then therapy for residual symptoms is administered according to the guidelines for treatment of functional psychosis presented in Chapter 6.

ORGANIC ANXIETY SYNDROME

Organic anxiety syndrome is diagnosed according to criteria presented in Table 7-9. Common etiologic factors associated with organic anxiety syndrome are listed in Table 6-5.

Treatment of organic anxiety syndrome is similar to treatment of organic mood syndrome and organic psychosis, that is, removal of potential exogenous causes and amelioration of potential endogenous causes is followed by treatment of residual anxiety with the appropriate combination of psychosocial and somatic therapies, as outlined in Chapter 6. Of the etiologies listed, one of the most avoidable and potentially dangerous is that associated

TABLE 7-9. **Diagnostic criteria for organic anxiety syndrome**

A. Prominent, recurrent, panic attacks or generalized anxiety

B. There is evidence from the history, physical examination, or laboratory tests of a specific organic factor (or factors) judged to be etiologically related to the disturbance.

C. Not occurring exclusively during the course of delirium.

Source. Adapted with permission from American Psychiatric Association: Diagnostic and Statistical Manual of Mental Disorders, 3rd Edition, Revised. Washington, DC, American Psychiatric Association, 1987, p 114. Copyright 1987 The American Psychiatric Association.

with withdrawal of central nervous system depressants. Because of the many advantages associated with short-acting as opposed to long-acting benzodiazepines, the former are widely prescribed for elderly patients. It is very important to instruct patients and spouses about the risks of sudden withdrawal, particularly if they have had past experience with longer-acting agents such as diazepam and have come to believe that abrupt discontinuation is painless and safe.

■ PSYCHOLOGICAL FACTORS AFFECTING PHYSICAL ILLNESS

DIRECT INFLUENCES

The well-known relationship between psychological factors and the development and exacerbation of physical illness holds among elderly patients as much, if not more, than among middle-aged patients. Any circumstance that leads to an increase in anxiety, anger, or depression is liable to be reflected in acute exacerbation of preexisting physical illness. Although almost any condition can be so affected, the more common geriatric illnesses are listed in Table 7-10. These conditions are so regularly exacerbated by fluctuations in anxiety, anger, or depression that acute, otherwise unexplained worsening in any of these illnesses may be a clue that the associated anxiety disorder, depressive disorder, or hypomanic-manic or paranoid disorder is undertreated.

MANAGING CHRONIC PAIN

Many of the most common medical illnesses of elderly patients produce chronic or intermittent pain that can be exacerbated by anxiety or depression. Also, for many elderly people, complaints of pain are seen as the most effective or acceptable way to gain attention from family members. Proper management of chronic pain therefore entails treatment of coexisting psychiatric illness and assessment of social support networks, in addition to careful regulation of analgesics. Some elderly patients can also benefit from behaviorally oriented pain management training, including relaxation techniques; patients free of significant memory prob-

TABLE 7-10. **Physical illnesses commonly exacerbated by psychological factors**

Anxiety commonly exacerbates:

- Acute pain
- Angina pectoris [a]
- Benign arrythmia [a]
- Chronic obstructive pulmonary disease, especially asthma
- Chronic pain
- Dermatitis
- Gastrointestinal dysfunction, including
    Dysphagia [a]
    Gastritis [a]
    "Irritable bowel syndrome" [a]
    Obesity
    Peptic ulcer [a]
    Vomiting
- Hypertension [a]
- Tension headache [a]
- Tardive and other dyskinesias
- Urinary hesitancy, frequency, urgency, or incontinence secondary to bladder infection or spasm

Depression commonly exacerbates:

- Chronic pain of any etiology, especially musculoskeletal
- Constipation
- Hypokinesia of Parkinson's disease
- Loss of energy, any cause
- Weakness, any cause

[a] Condition also commonly exacerbated by anger.

lems, with some insight into the synergistic effects of mood state on pain, are good candidates for such interventions.

INDIRECT INFLUENCES

Physical illnesses are subject to indirect influences of psychological states as well. Perhaps the most common and most hazardous such influence is failure to comply with treatment, either by failure to report new or worsening symptomatology or by failure to follow instructions regarding diet, activity, or medications. Among elderly psychiatric patients, major depression is commonly accompanied by passive refusal to attend to physical illness and by medication noncompliance. Forgetfulness associated with dementia may similarly contribute to missed appointments and under- or overdosage of prescribed medications and to potentially hazardous medication combinations. Psychoactive medication noncompliance among paranoid patients is almost the rule, whereas overuse of psychoactive and nonpsychoactive medications is common among substance abusers and hypomanic-manic patients.

Unfortunately, there are no useful guidelines in this area other than good clinical judgment and the willingness to enlist family, spouses, and board-and-care and nursing-home operators in the task of monitoring and encouraging compliance. Routine determination of serum levels of antidepressants and certain neuroleptics may also be of value in this context. Monoamine oxidase inhibitors pose a particular problem in this regard, as they are often the treatment of choice for the depressed-demented patient who is unfortunately at particular risk for inadvertent ingestion of sympathomimetic "cold pills" or dextromethorphan-containing cough remedies. Our policy is to only prescribe monoamine oxidase inhibitors when a cognitively intact, alert, and involved family member or spouse is in the household and commits to monitoring this important aspect of the treatment plan.

■ INFLUENCE OF AGING ON DISORDERS OF EARLY ONSET

MOOD DISORDERS

As described in Chapter 4, some differences in presentation of major depression in late life have been reported. In general, populations on which these observations are based were not selected for late onset, so the observed differences are likely to hold for early-onset disorders as well. Among aging patients with bipolar mood disorder, a tendency of the condition to "burn out" over time has been observed (13), whereas those who do not "burn out" tend to have more frequent and longer episodes and more rapid cycling (14). However, studies in this area are few and the data base for these generalizations leaves room for question.

SCHIZOPHRENIA

Little is known about the later stages of schizophrenia beyond a general impression that "positive" symptoms (hallucinations, bizarre behavior, agitation) tend to "burn out" and "negative" symptoms (passivity, withdrawal, anhedonia) come to dominate the clinical picture. It is not clear whether this development is related to the natural history of the disorder only or is significantly exacerbated by the debilitating effects of chronic neuroleptic therapy (15) and the impoverished environments in which most chronic schizophrenic patients grow old.

PERSONALITY DISORDERS

Few data have been gathered on Axis II disorders in elderly patients, in part because most of the personality disorders in DSM-III-R have not been defined long enough for thorough studies to have taken place. The only exception is antisocial personality disorder, which has been defined similarly for a long time. Here, it is well established that age is "curative" in the sense that the disorder almost disappears in middle-age and is rarely diagnosed after age 65. The natural process of burnout that has been postulated to account for this declining prevalence appears to operate in certain other personality disorders as well. In our experience with several thousand elderly inpatients, vivid descriptions of borderline, narcissistic, hysterical, and histrionic traits in medical records of long-past hospitalizations are rarely matched by behavior in the present. Moreover, information provided by spouses, relatives, and family physicians generally confirms the impression of significant "blunting" of disturbing personality traits with the passage of time. On the other hand, passive-aggressive, passive-dependent, schizoid, avoidant, and paranoid traits appear to survive the aging process quite well and in some cases seem to have worsened. However, it is clear that systematic research will be needed to confirm these informal clinical generalizations.

■ REFERENCES

1. American Psychiatric Association: Diagnostic and Statistical Manual of Mental Disorders, 3rd Edition, Revised. Washington, DC, American Psychiatric Association, 1987

2. Hauri PJ: Primary insomnia, in Treatments of Psychiatric Disorders: A Task Force Report of the American Psychiatric Association, Vol 3. Washington, DC, American Psychiatric Association, 1989, pp 2424–2433

3. Robbins LN, Helzer JE, Weissman MM, et al: Lifetime prevalence of specific psychiatric disorders in three sites. Arch Gen Psychiatry 41:949–958, 1984

4. Regier DA, Boyd JH, Burke JD Jr, et al: One month prevalence of mental disorders in the United States. Arch Gen Psychiatry 45:977–986, 1988

5. American Psychiatric Association: Diagnostic and Statistical Manual of Mental Disorders, 3rd Edition. Washington, DC, American Psychiatric Association, 1980

6. Hurt RD, Finlayson RE, Morse RM, et al: Alcoholism in elderly persons: medical aspects and prognosis of 216 inpatients. Mayo Clin Proc 63:753–760, 1988

7. Finlayson RE, Hurt RD, Davis LJ Jr, et al: Alcoholism in elderly persons: a study of the psychiatric and psychosocial features of 216 inpatients. Mayo Clin Proc 63:761–768, 1988

8. Mishara BL, Kastenbaum R: Alcohol and Old Age. New York, Grune & Stratton, 1980

9. Whitcup SM, Miller F: Unrecognized drug dependence in psychiatrically hospitalized elderly patients. J Am Geriatr Soc 35:297–301, 1987

10. Whitlock FA: Symptomatic Affective Disorder. New York, Academic, 1982

11. Benson DF, Blumer D (eds): Psychiatric Aspects of Neurologic Disease. New York, Grune & Stratton, 1975

12. Plotkin DA: Organic delusional syndrome and organic hallucinosis, in Treatments of Psychiatric Disorders: A Task Force Report of the American Psychiatric Association, Vol 2. Washington, DC, American Psychiatric Association, 1989, pp 831–839

13. Winokur G: The Iowa 500: heterogeneity and course in manic-depressive illness (bipolar). Compr Psychiatry 16:125–131, 1975

14. Cutler NR, Post RM: Life course of illness in untreated manic-depressive patients. Compr Psychiatry 23:101–115, 1982

15. Van Putten T, Spar JE: The board and care home: does it deserve a bad press? Hosp Community Psychiatry 30:461–464, 1979

■ ADDITIONAL READINGS

Abrams RC, Alexopoulos GS: Substance abuse in the elderly: over the counter and illegal drugs. Hosp Community Psychiatry 39:822–829, 1988

Beers M, Avorn J, Soumerai SB, et al: Psychoactive medication use in intermediate care facility residents. JAMA 260:3016–3020, 1988

Dagon EM: Sexuality and sexual dysfunction in the elderly, in Essentials of Geriatric Psychiatry. Edited by Lazarus LW, Jarvik LF, Foster JR, et al. New York, Springer, 1988, pp 41–65

Sturgis ET, Dolce JJ, Dickerson PC: Pain management in the elderly, in Handbook of Clinical Gerontology. Edited by Carstensen LL, Ededstein BA. New York, Pergamon, 1987, pp 190–204

INDEX

4481